Second Edition

Quick Medical Spanish

Peter Thomas Rogers, MD
Brigham and Women's Hospital Clinical Fellow
Vascular and Inverventional Radiology
Harvard Medical School
Boston, Massachusetts

Olga Ruiz-Rogers, MSW
Formerly of University of Chicago
and Cook County Hospital
Chicago, Illinois

APPLETON & LANGE
Stamford, Connecticut

97 98 99 00 01 / 10 9 8 7 6 5 4 3 2 1

Prentice Hall International (UK) Limited, *London*
Prentice Hall of Australia Pty. Limited, *Sydney*
Prentice Hall Canada. Inc., *Toronto*
Prentice Hall Hispanoamericana, S.A., *Mexico*
Prentice Hall of India Private Limited, *New Delhi*
Prentice Hall of Japan, Inc., *Tokyo*
Simon & Schuster Asia Pte. Ltd., *Singapore*
Editora Prentice Hall do Brasil Ltda., *Rio de Janeiro*
Prentice Hall, *Upper Saddle River, New Jersey*

Library of Congress Cataloging-in-Publication Data
Rogers, Peter Thomas.
Quick medical Spanish / Peter Thomas Rogers, Olga Ruiz-Rogers. — 2nd ed.
p. cm.
ISBN 0-8385-8258-3 (Pbk : alk. paper)
1. Spanish language—Conversation and phrase books (for medical personnel) I. Ruiz-Rogers, Olga. II. Title.
[DLNM: 1. Medicine—phrases—Spanish. W 15 R728q 1997]
PC4120.M3R6 1997
468.3´421´02461—dc20
DNLM/DLC
for Library of Congress 96-31450

Acquisitions Editor: John Dolan
Production Editor: Sondra Greenfield
Designer: Janice Barsevich Bielawa

PRINTED IN THE UNITED STATES OF AMERICA

0-8385-8258-3
9 780838 582589 90000

CONTENTS

PREFACE

Quick Medical Spanish, second edition, was written to help English-speaking hospital personnel communicate better with Spanish-speaking patients. Patients will appreciate your attempts to communicate with them in their language, and it will help you to understand and comfort them.

Quick Medical Spanish is designed to be user friendly and incorporates the following features:

1. A unique format that parallels the patient's history and physical examination, making it easy to follow along when interviewing patients.
2. A listing of the Spanish question word equivalents for who? (quién), what? (qué), where? (dónde), why? (porqué) and when? (cuándo) with examples (see Appendix B). Now you can ask questions in Spanish.
3. Medical questions are structured to elicit answers that are easy to understand such as "yes/no," numerical responses, and other single-word or short-phrase replies.
4. Use of pronouns *he/she/you* so that the same words can be used to address a question to the patient or a family member.
5. Text is written in outline format with the table of contents on the cover. This makes information easily accessible.

Our experience has shown that this approach facilitates rapid learning and effective communication. However, all of these phrases will be understood immediately by your patients. *Quick Medical Spanish* was written while working at a hospital that serves a large Hispanic population.

The time you take to learn the material in *Quick Medical Spanish* will be well rewarded. You will be amazed at how much this exercise can help you communicate with your Spanish-speaking patients. Your efforts and interest will be obvious to them as soon as you use your Spanish. You'll see it in their smiles.

Good luck!

Peter T. Rogers
Olga Ruiz-Rogers

ACKNOWLEDGMENTS

I would like to express my appreciation to the many people who, either directly or indirectly, helped make this book possible, including: John Dolan, Eric Newman, Dr. Jim Gomez, Dr. David Toovy and Dr. Kathy Harris, Dr. William Wallace, Dr. Jorge Girotti, Marsha Davis, Dr. Rolando and Milagros Toyos, The Urban Health Program and Center for Hispanic Excellence at the University of Illinois Medical School, Nellie Clark, Barbara Karklins, Frank Sparks, Dr. Bernadette Gochiuco, Dr. Truman Anderson, Dr. Laura Loya, Dr. Alexander Lin, Dr. Camelia McGrath, Dr. Heidi Eklund, Dr. Demetria Soter, Dr. Nina Garces, Dr. Elizabeth Yoder, Dr. Gebeyu, Dr. Arvind Nehra, Joe Madden, Kelley Celmer, Dr. Chuck Kinder, Shi Young, Consuelo Garrido, The Hispanic Health Care Task Force Committee at Northwestern Memorial Hospital of Northwestern Medical School, Dr. Ralph Tamura, Shondra Morrow RN, Margarita Galvin RN, and the great obstetric sonographers at Northwestern Memorial Hospital: Beth Clark RDMS, Jody Kalbach RDMS, Carol Scharm RDMS, Laurie Melnyczuk RDMS, Kim Accettura RDMS, Leanne Lanascese RDMS, Natalie Carr DDS, Dr. Joe Introcaso, Dr. Santiago Rossi, Cookie Armstrong, Aida Giron, Anna Grenvich, Dr. Natalie Carr, Marianella Cuadrado, Dr. Kevin Hannon and Suzie Rogers-Hannon, Michael Jr. and Jody Rogers, Eduardo Alvarez, Maria Perreira, Dr. Carlitos Alvarez, Dr. Munchie Alvarez, Dr. Irma Ruiz, Dr. Chito Ruiz, and, of course, most of all my parents Dr. Michael and Olga Ruiz-Rogers.

Cassette produced by Fireworks Music Inc. Keith Hooper, Producer.

Music from the album Implosion by Fireworks Jazz Ensemble. The song is Azul Obscuro by Steve Hashimoto.

This album and others available through Fireworks Music Inc., c/o Keith Hooper, Executive Producer & oboist, 400 S. Green Street #310, Chicago, Illinois, 60607-3504. (312) 666-4084.

MEDICAL HISTORY
Section One

1. INTRODUCTIONS

1. Hi, I am Mrs. Miller the nurse	Hola, yo soy la Señora Miller, la enfermera	(oh-**lah**, yoh soy lah seh-**nyohr**-rah mee-lehr, lah ehn-fehr-**mehr**-rah)
2. Hi, I am Ms. Miller the nurse	Hola, yo soy la Señorita Miller, la enfermera	(oh-**lah,** yoh soy lah seh-nyohr-**ee**-tah mee-lehr, lah ehn-fehr-**mehr**-rah)
3. Hi, I am Mr. Miller the nurse	Hola, yo soy el Señor Miller, el enfermero	(oh-**lah**, yoh soy ehl seh-**nyohr** mee-lehr, el ehn-fehr-**mehr**-roh)
4. Hi, I am Dr. Miller (female)	Hola, yo soy la doctora Miller	(oh-**lah**, yoh soy lah dohk-**toh**-rah mee-lehr)
5. Hi, I am Dr. Miller (male)	Hola, yo soy el doctor Miller	(oh-**lah**, yoh soy lah dohk-**tohr** mee-lehr)
6. I am Mary Miller, a medical student	Yo soy María Miller, una estudiante de medicina	(yoh soy mah-**ree**-ah mee-lehr oon-ah ehs-too-dee-**ahn**-teh deh meh-dee-**see**-nah)
7. I am the physical therapist	Yo soy la terapista física	(yoh soy lah teh-rah-**pees**-tah **fees**-ee-kah)
8. I am the social worker	Yo soy la trabajadora social	(yoh soy lah trah-bah-hah-**dohr**-ah soh-see-**al**)
9. I am the dietician	Yo soy la dietista	(yoh soy lah dee-eh-**tees**-tah)
10. What is your name?	¿Cómo se llama?	(**koh**-moh seh **yah**-mah)
11. What is your first name?	¿Cuál es su primer nombre?	(koo-**ahl** ehs soo pree-**mehr** **nohm**-breh)
12. What is your last name?	¿Cuál es su apellido?	(koo-**ahl** ehs soo ah-peh-**yee**-doh)
13. Do you speak English?	¿Habla inglés?	(**ah**-blah een-**glehs**)

14. I only speak a little Spanish	Sólo hablo un poquito de Español	(**soh**-loh **ah**-blah oon poh-**kee**-toh deh ehs-pah-**nyohl**)
15. Please speak very slowly	Por favor hable muy despacio	(pohr fah-**vohr ah**-bleh moo-ee deh-**spah**-see-oh)
16. I need to ask you some questions	Necesito hacerle unas preguntas	(neh-seh-**see**-toh ah-**sehr**-leh oon-ahs preh-**goon**-tahs)
17. Please answer my questions slowly and briefly	Por favor conteste mis preguntas despacio y breve	(pohr fah-**vohr** kohn-**tehs**-teh mees preh-**goon**-tahs dehs-**pah**-see-oh ee **breh**-veh)
18. More slowly	Más despacio	(**mahs** dehs-**pah**-see-oh)
19. Say that again, please	Otra vez, por favor	(oh-trah **vehs** pohr fah-**vohr**)

2. IDENTIFYING DATA

1. How old are you?	¿Cuántos años tiene usted?	(koo-**ahn**-tohs **ah**-nyohs tee-**ehn**-eh oos-**tehd**)
2. What is your date of birth?	¿Cuál es su fecha de nacimiento?	(koo-**ahl** ehs soo **feh**-chah deh nah-see-mee-**ehn**-toh)
3. What is your address?	¿Cuál es su dirección?	(koo-**ahl** ehs soo dee-rehk-see-**ohn**)
4. What is the zip code?	¿Cuál es el código postal?	(koo-**ahl** ehs ehl **koh**-dee-joh pohs-**tahl**)
5. Do you have a telephone?	¿Tiene un teléfono?	(tee-**ehn**-eh oon teh-**leh**-fohn-oh)
6. What is your telephone number?	¿Cuál es su número de teléfono?	(koo-**ahl** ehs soo **noo**-mehr-oh deh teh-**leh**-foh-noh)
7. Please write it here	Por favor, escríbalo aquí	(pohr fah-**vohr** ehs-**kree**-bah-loh ah-**kee**)

8. Do you live alone?	¿Vive sólo?	(vee-veh **soh**-loh)
9. What persons live with you?	¿Quiénes personas viven con usted?	(kee-**ehn**-ehs pehr-**soh**-nahs **vee**-vehn kohn oos-**tehd**)
10. Is this the first time you have visited this hospital?	¿Es esta la primera vez qué ha visitado este hospital?	(ehs ehs-**tah** lah pree-**mehr**-ah vehs keh ah vee-see-**tah**-doh ehs-tah ohs-pee-**tahl**)
11. When was the last time you were here?	¿Cuándo fue la última vez que estuvo aquí?	(koo-**ahn**-doh foo-eh lah **ool**-tee-mah vehs keh ehs-**too**-voh ah-**kee**)
12. Do you work?	¿Trabaja?	(trah-**bah**-hah)
13. What type of work?	¿Qué tipo de trabajo?	(**keh** tee-poh deh trah-**bah**-hoh)
14. Please sign here	Por favor, firme aquí	(pohr fah-**vohr** **feer**-meh ah-**kee**)

3. CHIEF COMPLAINT & HISTORY OF PRESENT ILLNESS

1. How are you feeling?	¿Cómo se siente?	(**koh**-moh seh see-**ehn**-teh)
2. What symptom are you most concerned about (has you most preoccupied)?	¿Cuál síntoma le preocupa más?	(koo-**ahl** **seen**-toh-mah leh pre-oh-koo-pah **mahs**)
3. What is the most important problem?	¿Cuál es el problema más importante?	(koo-**ahl** ehs ehl proh-**bleh**-mah **mahs** eem-pohr-**tahn**-teh)
4. Since when have you had this symptom?	¿Desde cuándo tiene este síntoma?	(**dehs**-deh koo-**ahn**-doh tee-**ehn**-eh ehs-teh **seen**-toh-mah)
5. How many minutes?	¿Cuántos minutos?	(koo-**ahn**-tohs meen-**oo**-tohs)
6. How many hours?	¿Cuántas horas?	(koo-**ahn**-tas **ohr**-ahs)
7. How many days?	¿Cuántos días?	(koo-**ahn**-tas **dee**-ahs)

8.	How many weeks?	¿Cuántas semanas?	(koo-**ahn**-tas seh-**mahn**-ahs)
9.	How many months?	¿Cuántos meses?	(koo-**ahn**-tas **meh**-sehs)
10.	How many years?	¿Cuántos años?	(koo-**ahn**-tas **ah**-nyohs)
11.	Did you have it today?	¿Lo tuvo hoy?	(loh **too**-voh oy)
12.	Did you have it yesterday?	¿Lo tuvo ayer?	(loh **too**-voh eye-**ehr**)
13.	Did you have it yesterday morning?	¿Ayer por la mañana?	(eye-**ehr** pohr lah ma-**nyah**-nah)
14.	Did you have it yesterday afternoon?	¿Ayer por la tarde?	(eye-**ehr** pohr lah **tahr**-deh)
15.	Did you have it yesterday evening?	¿Ayer por la noche?	(eye-**ehr** pohr la **noh**-cheh)
16.	The day before yesterday?	¿Anteayer?	(ahn-teh-eye-**ehr**)
17.	How many times?	¿Cuántas veces?	(koo-**ahn**-tas **veh**-sehs)
18.	What makes it better?	¿Qué lo mejora?	(**keh** loh meh-**hohr**-ah)
19.	What makes it worse?	¿Qué lo empeora?	(**keh** loh ehm-peh-**ohr**-ah)
20.	Have you ever had this in the past?	¿Ha tenido este síntoma en el pasado?	(ah teh-**nee**-doh ehs-teh **seen**-toh-mah ehl pah-**sah**-doh)
21.	Do you have any other symptoms?	¿Tiene algunos otros síntomas?	(tee-**ehn**-eh ahl-**goon**-ohs oh-trohs **seen**-toh-mahs)

4. ALLERGIES

1.	Do you have any allergies to medicines or foods?	¿Tiene alergias a las medicinas o comidas?	(tee-**ehn**-eh ah-lehr-**hee**-ahs ah lahs meh-dee-**seen**-ahs oh koh-**mee**-dahs)
2.	Penicillin, sulfas, aspirin?	¿Penicilina, sulfas o aspirina?	(pehn-ee-see-**lee**-nah **sool**-fahs oh ahs-pee-**ree**-nah)

3. What happens?	¿Qué ocurre?	(**keh** oh-**koo**-reh)
4. Did you have difficulty breathing?	¿Tuvo dificultad al respirar?	(**too**-voh dee-fee-kool-**tahd** ahl rehs-peer-**ahr**)
5. Did you get a rash?	¿Tuvo una erupción?	(**too**-voh oon-ah eh-roop-see-**ohn**)

5. MEDICATION HISTORY

1. Are you taking any medicines?	¿Toma algunas medicinas?	(**toh**-mah ahl-**goo**-nahs meh-dee-**see**-nahs)
2. What medicines?	¿Qué medicinas?	(**keh** meh-dee-**see**-nahs)
3. Heart pills	Pastillas para el corazón	(pahs-**tee**-yahs pah-rah ehl kohr-ah-**sohn**)
4. Antianginals	Medicina para el dolor del pecho	(meh-dee-**see**-nah pah-rah ehl doh-**lohr** dehl **peh**-choh)
5. Ionotropic agents	Medicina para aumentar las contracciones del corazón	(meh-dee-**see**-nah pah-rah ah-oo-mehn-**tahr** lahs kohn-trahk-see-**ohn**-ehs dehl kohr-ah-**sohn**)
6. Antiarrhythmics	Medicinas para mejorar el ritmo del corazón	(meh-dee-**see**-nahs pah-rah meh-hohr-**ahr** ehl **reet**-moh dehl kohr-ah-**sohn**)
7. Digoxin	Digoxina	(dee-hohx-**ee**-nah)
8. Medicines for hypertension	Medicinas para la hipertensión	(meh-dee-**see**-nahs pah-rah lah ee-pehr-tehn-see-**ohn**)
9. Diuretics	Diuréticos, medicinas para orinar más	(dee-oor-**eh**-tee-kohs meh-dee-**see**-nahs pah-rah oh-ree-**nahr mahs**)

10.	Antibiotics	Antibióticos	(ahn-tee-bee-**oh**-tee-kohs)
11.	Insulin	Insulina	(een-soo-**lee**-nah)
12.	Anticoagulants	Anticoagulantes, medicina para evitar la formación de coágulos	(ahn-tee-koh-ah-goo-**lahn**-tehs meh-dee-**see**-nah pah-rah eh-vee-**tahr** lah fohr-mah-see-**ohn** de koh-**ah**-goo-lohs)
13.	Analgesics	Pastillas para calmar el dolor	(pah-**stee**-yahs pah-rah kahl-**mahr** ehl doh-**lohr**)
14.	Steroids	Esteroides	(ehs-tehr-oh-**ee**-dehs)
15.	Prednisone	Prednisona	(prehd-nee-**soh**-nah)
16.	Antacids	Antiácidos	(ahn-tee-**ah**-see-dohs)
17.	Laxatives	Laxantes	(lahx-**ahn**-tehs)
18.	Antihistamine	Antihistamínico	(ahn-tee-ees-teh-**meen**-ee-koh)
19.	Morphine	Morfina	(mohr-**fee**-nah)
20.	Nitroglycerin	Nitroglicerina	(nee-troh-glee-sehr-**ee**-nah)
21.	Aspirin	Aspirina	(ahs-peer-**ee**-nah)
22.	Sedative	Sedante	(seh-**dahn**-teh)
23.	Anticonvulsants	Medicina para las convulsiones	(meh-dee-**see**-nah pah-rah las koon-vool-see-**ohn**-ehs)
24.	Heparin	Heparina	(eh-pahr-**ee**-nah)
25.	Birth control pills	La píldora anticonceptiva	(lah **peel**-dohr-ah ahn-tee-kohn-seph-**tee**-vah)
26.	Antihyperlipemic	Una medicina para bajar el colesterol y los triglíceridos	(oon-ah meh-dee-**see**-nah pah-rah bah-**har** ehl koh-lehs-ter-**ohl** ee lohs tree-**glee**-sehr-ee-dohs)
27.	Vitamins	Vitaminas	(vee-tah-**mee**-nahs)
28.	Antiemetic	Una medicina para la náusea y vómitos	(oon-ah meh-dee-**see**-nah pah-rah lah **nah**-oo-see-eh ee **voh**-mee-tohs)

29. Do you have the bottles with you?	¿Tiene las botellas con usted?	(tee-**ehn**-eh lahs boh-**teh**-yahs kohn oos-**tehd**)
30. Please show me the bottles	Por favor, enséñeme las botellas	(pohr fah-**vohr** ehn-**seh**-nyeh-meh lahs boh-**teh**-yahs)

6. PAST SURGICAL HISTORY

1. Have you ever had any surgery?	¿Ha tenido algunas cirugías?	(ah teh-**nee**-doh ahl-**goon**-ahs see-roo-**hee**-ahs)
2. What type?	¿Qué tipo?	(**keh tee**-poh)
3. Gallbladder	Vesícula biliar	(veh-**see**-koo-laah bee-lee-**ahr**)
4. Appendix	El apéndice	(ehl ah-**pehn**-dee-seh)
5. Colon	El colon	(ehl **koh**-lohn)
6. Stomach	El estómago	(ehl eh-**stoh**-mah-goh)
7. Hernia	Hernia	(ehr-**nee**-ah)
8. Uterus/hysterectomy	El útero, histerectomía	(ehl **oo**-tehr-oh ees-tehr-ehk-toh-**mee**-ah)
9. Did you have any problems with excess bleeding?	¿Tuvo algunos problemas con hemorragia excesiva?	(**too**-voh ahl-**goo**-nohs proh-**bleh**-mahs kohn eh-mohr-ah-**hee**-ah ehx-seh-**see**-veh)

7. PAST MEDICAL HISTORY

1. Do you have or have you had HTN?	¿Tiene o ha tenido la presión alta?	(tee-**ehn**-eh oh ah teh-**nee**-doh lah preh-see-**ohn ahl**-tah)
2. Heart disease	Enfermedad del corazón	(ehn-fehr-meh-**dahd** del kohr-ah-**sohn**)

3. Myocardial infarction, "heart attack"	Infarto cardíaco,"ataqué del corazón"	(een-**fahr**-toh kahr-**dee**-ah-koh ah-tah-**keh** dehl kohr-ah-**sohn**)
4. Rheumatic fever	Fiebre reumática	(fee-**eh**-breh reh-oo-**mah**-tee-kah)
5. Asthma	Asma	(**ahs**-mah)
6. Emphysema	Enfisema	(ehn-fee-**seh**-mah)
7. Pnemonia	Neumonía	(neh-oo-moh-**nee**-ah)
8. TB	Tuberculosis	(too-behr-koo-**loh**-sees)
9. Anemia	Anemia	(ah-neh-**mee**-ah)
10. Stomach or duodenal ulcers	Ulceras del estómago o duodeno	(ool-**sehr**-ahs dehl ehs-**toh**-mah-goh oh doo-oh-**dehn**-oh)
11. Cancer	Cáncer	(**kahn**-sehr)
12. What type?	¿Qué tipo?	(**keh tee**-poh)
13. Arthritis	Artritis	(ahr-**tree**-tees)
14. Diabetes	Díabetes	(**dee**-ah-beh-tehs)
15. How many years?	¿Por cuántos años?	(pohr koo-**ahn**-tohs **ah**-nyohs)
16. Do you take insulin?	¿Toma insulina?	(**toh**-mah een-soo-**lee**-nah)
17. What is your usual dose?	¿Cuál es su dosis usualmente?	(koo-**ahl** ehs soo **doh**-sees oos-oo-ahl-**mehn**-teh)
18. Epilepsy	Epilepsia	(eh-pee-lehp-**see**-ah)
19. Stroke	Derrame cerebral	(deh-**rah**-meh sehr-eh-**brahl**)
20. Do you have any other diseases?	¿Tiene algunas otras enfermedades?	(tee-**ehn**-eh ahl-**goo**-nahs **oh**-trahs ehn-fehr-meh-**dah**-dehs)
21. When did you have your last tetanus shot?	¿Cuándo tuvo su última vacuna de tétano?	(koo-**ahn**-do **too**-voh soo **ool**-tee-mah vah-**koo**-nah deh **teh**-tahn-oh)

8. SOCIAL HISTORY

1. Are you married or single?	¿Está casado o soltero?	(ehs-**tah** kah-**sah**-doh oh sohl **teh**-roh)
2. Divorced or widowed?	¿Divorciado o Viudo?	(dee-vohr-see-**ah**-doh oh vee-**oo**-doh)
3. Do you live alone?	¿Vive sólo?	(**vee**-veh **soh**-loh)
4. What persons live with you?	¿Quiénes personas viven con usted?	(kee-**ehn**-ehs pehr-**soh**-nahs **vee**-vehn kohn oos-**tehd**)
5. Do you have any children?	¿Tiene hijos?	(tee-**ehn**-eh **ee**-hohs)
6. How many children?	¿Cuántos hijos?	(koo-**ahn**-tohs **ee**-hohs)
7. Do you drink alcohol?	¿Toma alcohol?	(**toh**-mah ahl-koh-**ohl**)
8. Beer, wine, or hard liquor?	¿Cerveza, vino, o bebidas fuertes?	(sehr-**veh**-sah, **vee**-noh, oh beh-**bee**-dahs foo-**ehr**-tehs)
9. Do you smoke cigarettes?	¿Fuma cigarillos?	(**foo**-mah see-gahr-**ee**-yohs)
10. How many packs a day?	¿Cuántos paquetes cada día?	(koo-**ahn**-tohs pah-**keh**-tehs **kah**-dah **dee**-ah)
11. For how many years?	¿Por cuántos años ha fumado?	(pohr koo-**ahn**-tohs **ah**-nyohs ah foo-**mah**-doh)
12. Do you use any drugs?	¿Usa algunas drogas?	(**oo**-sah ahl-**goo**-nahs **droh**-gahs)
13. Cocaine	Cocaína	(koh-kah-**ee**-nah)
14. Crack	Crack	(krahk)
15. Heroin	Heroína	(ehr-oh-**ee**-nah)
16. Have you ever had a test for AIDS?	¿Ha tenido alguna vez una prueba de SIDA?	(ah teh-**nee**-doh ahl-**goo**-nah vehs oo-nah proo-**eh**-bah deh **see**-dah)

17. Was it positive or negative?	¿Fue positivo o negativo?	(foo-eh poh-see-**tee**-voh oh neh-gah-**tee**-voh)

9. CHEST PAIN

1. Do you have chest pain?	¿Tiene dolor del pecho?	(tee-**ehn**-eh doh-**lohr** dehl **peh**-choh)
2. Show me where it hurts?	¿Enséñeme dónde le duele?	(ehn-**seh**-nyeh-meh **dohn**-deh leh doo-**eh**-leh)
3. How long does it last?	¿Cúanto tiempo duró?	(koo-**ahn**-toh tee-**ehm**-poh doo-**roh**)
4. What makes it worse?	¿Qué lo empeora?	(**keh** loh ehm-peh-**ohr**-ah)
5. Activity	Actividad	(ahk-tee-vee-**dahd**)
6. Walking	Caminar	(kah-mee-**nahr**)
7. Breathing	Respirar	(rehs-pee-**rahr**)
8. What makes it better?	¿Qué lo mejora?	(**keh** loh meh-**hohr**-ah)
9. Rest	Descanso	(dehs-**kahn**-soh)
10. Medicine	Medicina	(meh-dee-**see**-nah)
11. Is the pain sharp or dull?	¿Es el dolor agudo o sordo?	(ehs ehl doh-**lohr** ah-**goo**-doh oh **sohr**-doh)
12. Constant or intermittent	Constante o intermitente	(kohn-**stahn**-teh oh een-tehr-mee-**tehn**-teh)
13. Do you feel tightness in your chest?	¿Siente el pecho apretado?	(see-**ehn**-teh ehl **peh**-choh al-preh-**tah**-doh)

14.	Mild, moderate, or severe?	¿Mínimo, moderado, o severo?	(**mee**-nee-moh, moh-dehr-**ah**-doh, oh seh-**vehr**-oh)
15.	Did you have palpitations?	¿Tuvo palpitaciones?	(**too**-voh pahl-pee-tah-see-**ohn**-ehs)
16.	Have you had this pain in the past?	¿Ha tenido este dolor en el pasado?	(ah teh-**nee**-doh ehs-teh doh-**lohr** ehn ehl pah-**sah**-doh)
17.	Cardiac Care Unit	La sala de cuidado cardíaco	(lah **sah**-lah deh koo-ee-**dah**-doh cahr-**dee** ah-koh)
18.	Intensive Care Unit	La sala de cuidado intensivo	(lah **sah**-lah deh koo-ee-**dah**-doh een-tehn-**see**-voh)
19.	Pacemaker	Marcapaso	(mahr-kah-**pah**-soh)
20.	Have you ever had a heart attack?	¿Ha tenido alguna vez un ataque al corazón?	(ah teh-**nee**-doh ahl-**goo**-nah vehs oon ah-tah-**keh** ahl kohr-ah-**sohn**)
21.	Myocardial Infarction	Infarto cardíaco	(een-**fahr**-toh kahr-**dee**-ah-koh)
22.	Have you ever had a cardiac arteriogram?	¿Ha tenido alguna vez un arteriograma del corazón?	(ah teh-**nee**-doh ahl-**goo**-nah vehs oon ahr-tehr-ee-oh-**grah**-mah dehl kohr-ah-**sohn**)
23.	Did you have nausea or vomiting?	¿Tuvo náusea o vómitos?	(too-voh **nah**-oo-seh-ah oh **voh**-mee-tohs)
24.	Does the pain move to your arm or jaw?	¿Se extiende dolor a su brazo o mandíbula?	(seh ehx-tee-**ehn**-deh doh-**lohr** ah soo **brah**-soh oh mahn-**dee**-boo-lah)
25.	Did you sweat a lot?	¿Tuvo mucho sudor?	(**too**-voh **moo**-choh soo-**dohr**)
26.	In your face or forehead?	¿En la cara o frente?	(ehn lah **kah**-rah oh **frehn**-teh)
27.	Congestive heart failure?	¿Insuficiencia cardíaca congestiva?	(een-soo-fee-see-**ehn**-see-ah kahr-**dee**-ah-kah kohn-heh-**stee**-vah)

10. ABSOLUTE AND RELATIVE CONTRAINDICATIONS TO THROMBOLYSIS (A PARTIAL LIST)

1. Have you had blood in your stool or urine in the past 10 days?	¿Ha tenido sangre en el excremento u orina en los pasados diez días?	(ah teh-**nee**-doh **sahn**-greh ehn ehl ehx-creh-**mehn**-toh oo oh-**ree**-nah ehn lohs pah-**sah**-dohs dee-ehs **dee**-ahs)
2. Have you had surgery or a biopsy in the past 10 days?	¿Ha tenido cirugía o una biopsia en los pasados diez días?	(Ah teh-**nee**-doh see-roo-**hee**-ah oh oon-ah bee-ohp-**see**-ah ehn lohs pah-**sah**-dohs dee-ehs **dee**-ahs)
3. Have you had a major trauma recently?	¿Ha tenido un traumatismo severo?	(ah teh-**nee**-doh oon trah-oo-mah-**tees**-moh seh-**vehr**-oh)
4. Do you have a brain tumor or arteriovenous malformation?	¿Tiene un tumor del cerebro o una malformación arteriovenosa?	(tee-**ehn**-eh oon too-**mohr** dehl seh-**reh**-broh oh oon-ah mahl-fahr-mah-see-**ohn** ahr-tehr-ee-oh-vehn-**oh**-sah)
5. Have you had brain surgery during the past 2 months?	¿Ha tenido cirugía del cerebro durante los pasados dos meses?	(ah teh-**nee**-doh see-roo-**hee**-ah-dehl seh-**reh**-broh doo-**rahn**-teh lohs pah-**sah**-dohs dohs **meh**-sehs)
6. Have you had a stroke, or TIA during the past 12 months?	¿Ha tenido un derrame cerebral o ataqué isqémico transitorio durante los doce meses pasado?	(ah teh-**nee**-doh oon deh-**rah**-meh seh-reh-**brahl** oh ah-tah-**keh** ees-**kehm**-ee-koh trahn-see-tohr-**ee**-oh doo-rahn-teh lohs **doh**-seh **meh**-sehs pah-**sah**-doh)
7. Do you have a heart infection?	¿Tiene un infección del corazón?	(tee-**ehn**-eh oon een-fehk-see-**ohn** dehl kohr-ah-**sohn**)

8. Are you pregnant?	¿Está embarazada?	(ehs-**tah** ehm-bah-rah-**sah**-dah)
9. When was your last menstrual period?	¿Cuándo fue su última regla?	(koo-**ahn**-doh foo-eh soo **ool**-tee-mah **reh**-glah)

11. GASTROINTESTINAL DISEASES

1. Do you have abdominal pain?	¿Tiene dolor en su abdomen?	(tee-ehn-eh doh-**lohr** ehn soo ahb-**doh**-mehn)
2. Show me where it hurts the most with one finger	Enséñeme donde le duele más con un dedo	ehn-**seh**-nyeh-meh **dohn**-deh leh doo-eh-leh **mahs** kohn oon **deh**-doh)
3. Does it hurt here?	¿Le duele aquí?	(leh doo-eh-leh ah-**kee**)
4. How long have you had this pain?	¿Desde cuándo tiene este dolor?	(dehs-deh koo-**ahn**-doh tee-**eh**-neh ehs-teh doh-**lohr**)
5. Do you have nausea or vomiting?	¿Tiene náusea o vómitos?	(tee-ehn-eh **nah**-oo-seh-ah oh **voh**-mee-tohs)
6. Do you have diarrhea?	¿Tiene díarrea?	(tee-**ehn**-eh **dee**-ahr-eh-ah)
7. Do you have constipation?	¿Tiene estreñimiento?	(tee-**ehn**-eh ehs-trehn-ee-mee-**ehn**-toh)
8. When was your last bowel movement?	¿Cuándo fue su último excremento?	(koo-**ahn**-doh foo-eh soo **ool**-tee-moh ehx-creh-**mehn**-toh)
9. Do you have blood in your stools?	¿Tiene sangre en los excrementos?	(tee-**ehn**-eh sahn-greh ehn lohs ehx-creh-**mehn**-tohs)
10. What makes it worse?	¿Qué lo empeora?	(**keh** loh ehm-peh-**ohr**-ah)
11. What makes it better?	¿Qué lo mejora?	(**keh** loh meh-**hohr**-ah)

12.	Have you been drinking?	¿Ha tomado alcohol?	(ah toh-**mah**-doh ahl-koh-**ohl**)
13.	Beer, wine, or hard liquor?	¿Cerveza, vino o bebidas fuertes?	(sehr-**veh**-sah **vee**-noh oh beh-**bee**-dahs foo-**ehr**-tehs)
14.	When was your last meal?	¿Cuándo fue su última comida?	(koo-**ahn**-doh foo-eh soo **ool**-tee-mah koh-**mee**-dah)
15.	Are you hungry now?	¿Tiene hambre ahora?	(tee-**ehn**-eh **ahm**-breh ah-**ohr**-ah)
16.	Have you ever had an U/S of your gallbladder?	¿Ha tenido alguna vez un ultrasonido de la vesícula biliar?	(ah teh-**nee**-doh ahl-**goo**-nah vehs oon ool-trah-soh-**nee**-doh deh lah veh-**see**-koo-lah bee-lee-**ahr**)
17.	When?	¿Cuándo?	(koo-**ahn**-doh)
18.	Did you have gallstones?	¿Tuvo cálculos?	(too-voh **kahl**-koo-lohs)
19.	Do you have hepatitis?	¿Tiene hepatitis?	(tee-**ehn**-eh eh-pah-**tee**-tees)

12. SHORTNESS OF BREATH

1.	Are you short of breath?	¿Tiene falta de aire?	(tee-**ehn**-eh **fahl**-tah deh **ahr**-eh)
2.	Are you having difficulty breathing?	¿Tiene dificultad al respirar?	(tee-**ehn**-eh dee-fee-kool-**tahd** ahl rehs-peer-**ahr**)
3.	Since when?	¿Desde cuándo?	(**dehs**-deh koo-**ahn**-doh)
4.	Do you have asthma?	¿Tiene asma?	(tee-**ehn**-eh **ahs**-mah)
5.	Do you have emphysema?	¿Tiene enfisema?	(tee-**ehn**-eh ehn-fee-**seh**-mah)
6.	Have you had a fever?	¿Ha tenido fiebre?	(ah teh-**nee**-doh fee-**eh**-breh)
7.	Have you had a cough?	¿Ha tenido tos?	(ah teh-**nee**-doh tohs)

8. Have you ever had this in the past?	¿Ha tenido esto en el pasado?	(ah teh-**nee**-doh **ehs**-toh ehn ehl pah-**sah**-doh)
9. What makes it better?	¿Qué lo mejora?	(**keh** loh meh-**hohr**-ah)
10. Rest, inhalers, or steroids?	¿Descanso, inhaladores, o esteroides?	(dehs-**kahn**-soh, een-hahl-ah-**dohr**-ehs, oh ehs-tehr-oh-**ee**-dehs)
11. What makes it worse?	¿Qué lo empeora?	(**keh** loh ehm-peh-**ohr**-ah)
12. Activity, walking, or lying flat	Actividad, caminar, o acostarse	(ahk-tee-vee-**dahd**, kah-mee-**nahr**, oh ah-koh-**stahr**-seh)
13. Do your ankles sometimes swell?	¿Se le hinchan los tobillos?	(seh leh **een**-chahn lohs toh-**bee**-yohs)
14. Have you ever needed to be hospitalized for this condition?	¿Ha necesitado hospitalización para esta condición?	(ah neh-seh-see-**tah**-doh ohs-pee-tahl-ee-sah-see-**ohn** pah-rah ehs-tah kohn-dee-see-**ohn**)
15. Have you ever needed to be intubated?	¿Ha necesitado intubación?	(ah neh-seh-see-**tah**-doh een-too-bah-see-**ohn**)

13. GENITOURINARY DISEASES

1. Have you ever had kidney stones?	¿Ha tenido alguna vez cálculos en los riñones?	(ah teh-**nee**-doh ahl-**goo**-nah vehs **kahl**-koo-lohs ehn lohs ree-**nyoh**-nehs)
2. Did the pain start gradually or rapidly?	¿Empieza el dolor rápido o gradualmente?	(ehm-pee-**eh**-sah ehl doh-**lohr** **rah**-pee-doh oh grah-doo-ahl-**mehn**-teh)
3. Show me where it hurts	Enséñeme donde le duele	(ehn-**seh**-nyeh-meh **dohn**-deh leh doo-**eh**-leh)

4. Does the pain radiate?	¿Se extiende el dolor?	(seh ehx-tee-**ehn**-deh ehl doh-**lohr**)
5. From where to where?	¿De dónde a dónde?	(deh **dohn**-deh ah **dohn**-deh)
6. Do you have blood in your urine?	¿Tiene sangre en la orina?	(tee-**ehn**-eh **sahn**-greh ehn lah oh-**ree**-nah)
7. Do you have nausea?	¿Tiene náusea?	(tee-**ehn**-eh **nah**-oo-seh-ah)
8. Do you have or have you had problems with:	¿Tiene o ha tenido problemás con:	(tee-**ehn**-eh oh ah teh-**nee**-doh proh-bleh-**mahs** kohn)
9. Kidneys?	¿Los riñones?	(lohs ree-**nyoh**-nehs)
10. Bladder?	¿La vejiga?	(lah veh-**hee**-gah)
11. Prostate?	¿La próstata?	(lah **prohs**-tah-tah)
12. Do you have difficulty urinating?	¿Tiene dificultad al orinar?	(tee-**ehn**-eh dee-fee-kool-**tahd** ahl oh-ree-**nahr**)
13. How many times did you urinate today?	¿Cuántas veces orinó hoy?	(koo-**ahn**-tahs **veh**-sehs oh-ree-**noh** oy)
14. Yesterday	Ayer	(eye-**ehr**)

14. SEXUALLY TRANSMITTED DISEASES

1. Do you have or have you had?	¿Tiene o ha tenido?	(tee-**ehn**-eh oh ah teh-**nee**-doh)
2. Herpes	Herpes	(**ehr**-pehs)
3. Gonorrhea	Gonorrea	(goh-nohr-**eh**-ah)
4. Syphilis	Sífilis	(**see**-fee-lees)

5. Condyloma, genital warts	Condiloma, verrugas genitales	(kohn-dee-**loh**-mah, veh-**roo**-gahs heh-nee-**tahl**-ehs)
6. Did you have treatment?	¿Tuvo tratamiento?	(too-voh trah-tah-mee-**ehn**-toh)
7. What treatment?	¿Qué tipo de tratamiento?	(**keh** tee-poh deh trah-tah-mee-**ehn**-toh)
8. For how long?	¿Cuánto duró el tratamiento?	(koo-**ahn**-toh doo-**roh** ehl trah-tah-mee-**ehn**-toh)
9. Do you have pain or burning when you urinate?	¿Tiene dolor o ardor Cuándo orina?	(tee-**ehn**-eh doh-**lohr** oh ahr-**dohr** koo-ahn-doh oh-**ree**-nah)

15. DIABETES

1. Do you have diabetes?	¿Tiene díabetes?	(tee-**ehn**-eh **dee**-ah-beh-tehs)
2. How many years?	¿Por cuántos años?	(pohr koo-**ahn**-tohs **ah**-nyohs)
3. Do you take insulin?	¿Ha tomado insulina?	(ah toh-**mah**-doh een-soo-**lee**-nah)
4. When was your last dose?	¿Cuándo fue su última dósis?	(koo-**ahn**-doh **foo**-eh soo **ool**-tee-mah **doh**-sees)
5. When was your last meal?	¿Cuándo fue su última comidas?	(koo-**ahn**-doh **foo**-eh soo **ool**-tee-mah koh-**mee**-dahs)
6. Did you ever lose consciousness?	¿Ha perdido alguna vez el conocimiento?	(ah per-**dee**-doh ahl-**goon**-ah vehs ehl koh-noh-see-mee-**ehn**-toh)
7. Are you taking any other medicines for your diabetes?	¿Toma algunas otras medicinas para la díabetes?	(toh-mah ahl-**goo**-nahs oh-trahs meh-dee-**see**-nahs pah-rah lah **dee**-ah-beh-tehs)

16. RASH

1. Do you have a rash?	¿Tiene una erupción?	(tee-**ehn**-eh oon-ah eh-roop-see-**ohn**)
2. Where is the rash?	¿Dónde está la erupción?	(**dohn**-deh ehs-**tah** lah eh-roop-see-**ohn**)
3. Does it itch?	¿Tiene picazón?	(tee-**ehn**-eh pee-kah-**sohn**)
4. Do not scratch it	No se rasque	(no seh **rahs**-keh)

17. FEVER

1. How many days have you had a fever?	¿Por cuántos días ha tenido fiebre?	(pohr koo-**ahn**-tahs **dee**-ahs ah teh-**nee**-doh fee-**eh**-breh)
2. What was the temperature?	¿Cuál fue la temperatura?	(koo-**ahl** foo-eh lah tehm-pehr-ah-**too**-rah)
3. Do you have a thermometer?	¿Tiene un termómetro?	(tee-**ehn**-eh oon tehr-**moh**-meh-troh)
4. Did you just touch your forehead?	¿Solamente tocó la frente?	(soh-lah-**mehn**-teh toh-**koh** lah **frehn**-teh)
5. Was it very hot?	¿Estaba muy caliente?	(ehs-**tah**-bah moo-ee kah-lee-**ehn**-teh)
6. Was it only a little hot?	¿Estaba solamente un poco caliente?	(ehs-**tah**-bah soh-lah-**mehn**-teh oon poh-koh kah-lee-**ehn**-teh)
7. Do you have a headache?	¿Tiene dolor de cabeza?	(tee-**ehn**-eh doh-**lohr** deh kah-**beh**-sah)

8. Does your neck feel stiff?	¿Se siente el cuello rígido?	(seh see-**ehn**-teh ehl koo-**eh**-yoh **ree**-jee-doh)
9. Do you have nausea?	¿Tiene náusea?	(tee-**ehn**-eh **nah**-oo-seh-ah)
10. Did you vomit?	¿Tuvo vómitos?	(too-voh **voh**-mee-tohs)
11. With a lot of mucus or phlegm?	¿Con mucho moco o flema?	(kohn **moo**-choh moh-koh oh **fleh**-mah)
12. What color?	¿De qué color?	(deh **keh** koh-**lohr**)
13. Grey, white, yellow, green?	¿Gris, blanco, amarillo, o verde?	(grees, **blahn**-koh, ah-mah-**ree**-yoh, oh **vehr**-deh)
14. Do you have a cough?	¿Tiene tos?	(tee-**ehn**-eh tohs)
15. Did you have chills?	¿Tuvo escalofríos?	(too-voh ehs-kah-loh-**free**-ohs)
16. Have you taken any tylenol or aspirin?	¿Ha tomado algún tylenol o aspirina?	(ah toh-mah-doh ahl-**goon** tee-leh-**nohl** o ahs-peer-**ee**-nah)
17. Do you have night sweats?	¿Tiene mucho sudor en la noche?	(tee-**ehn**-eh moo-choh soo-**dohr** ehn lah **noh**-cheh)
18. Does anyone else have the same symptoms?	Alguna otra persona tiene los mismos síntomás	(ahl-**goo**-nah oh-trah pehr-**soh**-nah tee-**ehn**-eh lohs **mees**-mohs **seen**-toh-mahs)

18. HEADACHE

1. Do you have a headache (HA)?	¿Tiene dolor de cabeza?	(tee-**ehn**-eh doh-**lohr** deh kah-**beh**-sah)
2. Is this the worst HA of your life?	¿Es este dolor de cabeza el peor de su vida?	(ehs ehs-teh doh-**lohr** deh kah-**beh**-sah ehl peh-**ohr** deh soo **vee**-dah)

3. Point to where it hurts	Enséñeme dónde le duele	(ehn-**seh**-nyeh-meh **dohn**-deh leh doo-**eh**-leh)
4. Have you had HAs in the past?	¿Ha tenido dolores de cabeza en el pasado?	(ah teh-**nee**-doh doh-**lohr**-ehs deh kah-**beh**-sah oh ehl pah-**sah**-doh)
5. When do you have HAs?	¿Cuándo tiene dolores de cabeza?	(koo-**ahn**-doh tee-**ehn**-eh doh-**lohr**-ehs deh kah-**beh**-sah)
6. In the morning?	¿En la mañana?	(ehn lah mah-**nyah**-nah)
7. In the afternoon?	¿En la tarde?	(ehn lah **tahr**-deh)
8. In the evening?	¿En la noche?	(ehn lah **noh**-cheh)
9. How many times per week?	¿Cuántas veces en una semana?	(koo-**ahn**-tahs veh-sehs ehn oon-ah seh-**mahn**-ah)
10. How many times per month?	¿Cuántas veces en un mes?	(koo-**ahn**-tahs veh-sehs ehn oon **mehs**)
11. How long does it last?	¿Cuánto tiempo dura?	(koo-**ahn**-toh tee-**ehm**-poh **doo**-rah)
12. Do you also have nausea and vomiting?	¿Tiene náusea o vómitos?	(tee-**ehn**-eh **nah**-oo-seh-ah oh **voh**-mee-tohs)

19. SYNCOPE

1. Did you (or he/she) faint?	¿Tuvo un desmayo?	(too-voh oon dehs-**meye**-oh)
2. Did you (or he/she) lose consciousness?	¿Perdió el conocimiento?	(pehr-dee-**oh** ehl koh-noh-seh-mee-**ehn**-toh)
3. For how long?	¿Por cuánto tiempo?	(pohr koo-**ahn**-toh tee-**ehm**-poh)

4. Did you have palpitations?	¿Tiene palpitaciones?	(tee-**ehn**-eh pahl-pee-tah-see-**ohn**-ehs)
5. Do you feel dizzy?	¿Tiene mareos?	(tee-**ehn**-eh mah-**reh**-ohs)
6. Do you have any other medical diseases?	¿Tiene algunas otras enfermedades?	(tee-**ehn**-eh ahl-**goo**-nahs oh-trahs ehn-fehr-meh-**dah**-dehs)
7. What medicines are you taking?	¿Qué medicinas toma?	(**keh** meh-dee-**see**-nahs **toh**-mah)

20. SEIZURES

1. Do you have epilepsy?	¿Tiene epilepsia?	(tee-**ehn**-eh eh-pee-lehp-**see**-ah)
2. Have you ever had these symptoms before?	¿Ha tenido alguna vez estos síntomás?	(ah ten-**nee**-doh ahl-**goo**-nah vehs **ehs**-tohs seen-toh-**mahs**)
3. Did the whole body move or just a part?	¿Se movió todo el cuerpo o solamente una parte?	(seh moh-vee-**oh** toh-doh ehl koo-**ehr**-poh oh soh-lah-**mehn**-teh oon-ah **pahr**-teh)
4. What part?	¿Qué parte?	(**keh** par-teh)
5. What medicines are you taking?	¿Qué medicinas toma?	(**keh** meh-dee-**see**-nahs **toh**-mah)
6. Have you ever had a head injury?	¿Ha tenido alguna vez un golpe en la cabeza?	(ah teh-**nee**-doh ahl-**goo**-nah vehs oon **gohl**-peh ehn lah kah-**beh**-seh)
7. During the seizure (Sz) did he/she fall and hurt himself/herself?	¿Durante la convulsión, se cayó y se lastimó?	(doo-**rahn**-teh lah kohn-vool-see-**ohn** seh keye-**oh** ee seh lahs-tee-**moh**)
8. During the Sz did he urinate or defecate?	¿Perdió el control de la orina o excremento?	(pehr-dee-**oh** ehl kohn-**trohl** deh lah oh-**ree**-nah oh ehx-creh-**mehn**-toh)

21. CEREBROVASCULAR ACCIDENT

1. Have you ever had a stroke?	¿Ha tenido alguna vez un derrame cerebral?	(ah teh-**nee**-doh ahl-**goo**-nah vehs oon deh-**rah**-meh seh-reh-**brahl**)
2. Can you move your fingers?	¿Puede mover los dedos?	(poo-**eh**-deh moh-vehr lohs **deh**-dohs)
3. Squeeze my fingers	Apriete mis dedos	(ah-pree-**eh**-teh mees **deh**-dohs)
4. Can you move your toes?	¿Puede mover los dedos del pie?	(poo-**eh**-deh moh-vehr lohs **deh**-dohs dehl **pee**-eh)
5. Push	Empuje	(ehm-**poo**-heh)
6. Do you have any other diseases?	¿Tiene algunas otras enfermedades?	(tee-**ehn**-eh ahl-**goo**-nahs oh-trahs ehn-fehr-meh-**dah**-dehs)
7. What medicines are you taking?	¿Qué medicinas toma?	(**keh** meh-dee-**see**-nas **toh**-mah)
8. Do you have numbness or weakness in your arm or leg?	¿Tiene adormecido o débil su brazo o pierna?	(tee-**ehn**-eh ah-dohr-meh-**see**-doh oh **deh**-beel soo **brah**-soh oh pee-**ehr**-nah)
9. Did you lose your vision temporarily?	¿Perdió su visión temporalmente?	(pehr-dee-**oh** soo vee-see-**ohn** tehm-pohr-ahl-**mehn**-teh)

22. TRAUMA

1. A—Do you have any allergies?	¿Tiene algunas alergias?	(tee-**ehn**-eh ahl-**goo**-nahs ah-lehr-**hee**-ahs)

2. M—What medicines are you taking?	¿Qué medicinas toma?	(**keh** meh-dee-**see**-nahs **toh**-mah)
3. P—Do you have any diseases?	¿Tiene algunas enfermedades?	(tee-**ehn**-eh ahl-**goo**-nahs ehn-fehr-meh-**dah**-dehs)
4. L—When was your last meal?	¿Cuándo fue su última comida?	(koo-**ahn**-doh foo-eh soo **ool**-tee-mah koh-**mee**-dah)
5. E—What happened?	¿Qué occurió?	(**keh** oh-koo-ree-**oh**)
6. Did you lose consciousness?	¿Perdió el conocimiento?	(pehr-dee-**oh** ehl koh-noh-see-mee-**ehn**-toh)
7. Where does it hurt?	¿Dónde le duele?	(**dohn**-deh leh doo-**eh**-leh)
8. Does your neck hurt?	¿Tiene dolor en su cuello?	(tee-**ehn**-eh doh-**lohr** ehn soo koo-**eh**-yoh)
9. Do not move your head	No mueva su cabeza	(noh moo-**eh**-vah soo kah-**beh**-sah)
10. Does your back hurt?	¿Tiene dolor de espalda?	(tee-**ehn**-eh doh-**lohr** deh ehs-**pahl**-deh)
11. Have you ever had any surgery?	¿Ha tenido algunas cirugías?	(ah teh-**nee**-doh ahl-**goo**-nahs see-roo-**hee**-ahs)
12. Do you have any heart problems?	¿Tiene enfermedades del corazón?	(tee-**ehn**-eh ehn-fehr-meh-**dah**-dehs dehl kohr-ah-**sohn**)
13. Can you move your fingers?	¿Puede mover los dedos?	(poo-**eh**-deh moh-vehr los **deh**-dohs)
14. Can you move your toes?	¿Puede mover los dedos del pie?	(poo-**eh**-deh moh-vehr lohs **deh**-dohs dehl **pee**-eh)
15. I need to start an IV	Necesito comenzar una línea intravenosa	(neh-seh-**see**-toh koh-mehn-**sahr** oon-ah **lee**-ne-sh een-trah-vehn-**oh**-sah)
16. Have you been drinking?	¿Ha tomado alcohol?	(ah toh-**mah**-doh ahl-koh-**ohl**)

23. MINOR LACERATION

1.	You have a cut/wound	Tiene una herida	(tee-**ehn**-eh oon-ah ehr-**ee**-dah)
2.	We need to clean it	Necesitamos limpiarla	(neh-seh-see-**tah**-mos leem-pee-**ahr**-lah)
3.	This is an antiseptic	Esto es un antiséptico	(**ehs**-toh ehs oon ahn-tee-**sehp**-tee-koh)
4.	You will need some stitches	Necesitará algunos puntos	(neh-seh-see-tah-**rah** ahl-**goo**-nohs **poon**-tohs)
5.	I will give you a local anesthetic	Le daré anestesia local	(leh dahr-**eh** ahn-ehs-teh-**see**-ah loh-**kahl**)
6.	It will only hurt a little bit	Sólo le dolerá un poco	(**soh**-loh leh doh-lehr-**ah** oon **poh**-koh)
7.	This is an antibiotic ointment	Esto es una pomada antibiótica	(ehs-toh ehs oon-ah poh-**mah**-da ahn-tee-bee-**oh**-tee-koh)
8.	You need to take an antibiotic	Necesita tomar un antibiótico	(neh-seh-**see**-tah toh-**mahr** oon ahn-tee-bee-**oh**-tee-koh)
9.	You need to return to the emergency room (ER) in one week to have the stitches removed	Necesita regresar a la sala de emergencia en una semana para remover los puntos	(neh-seh-**see**-tah reh-greh-**sahr** ah lah **sah**-lah deh eh-mehr-hehn-**see**-ah ehn oon-ah seh-**mah**-nah pah-rah reh-moh-vehr lohs **poon**-tohs)
10.	When was your last tetanus shot?	¿Cuándo fue su última inyección de tétano?	(koo-**ahn**-doh foo-eh soo **ool**-tee-mah een-yehk-see-**ohn** deh **teh**-tahn-oh)
11.	You should have a tetanus shot now	Debe tener una vacuna de tétano ahora	(deh-beh teh-**nehr** oon-ah vah-**koon**-ah deh **teh**-tahn-oh ah-**ohr**-ah)

24. PERIPHERAL VASCULAR DISEASE

1.	Do you have pain in your leg?	¿Tiene dolor en su pierna?	(tee-**ehn**-eh doh-**lohr** ehn soo pee-**ehr**-nah)
2.	Right, left, or both?	¿Derecha, izquierda o ambas?	(dehr-**eh**-chah ees-kee-**ehr**-dah oh **ahm**-bahs)
3.	Which side is worse?	¿Cuál está peor?	(koo-**ahl** ehs-**tah** peh-**ohr**)
4.	Does the pain occur when you are walking?	¿Le occure cuándo camina?	(leh oh-**koo**-reh koo-**ahn**-doh kah-**mee**-nah)
5.	Is it always the same distance, approximately "more or less"?	¿Es siempre la misma distancia aproximadamente "más o menos"?	(ehs see-**ehm**-preh lah **mees**-mah dees-tahn-**see**-ah ah-prohx-ee-mah-dah-**mehn**-teh **mahs** oh **meh**-nohs)
6.	One or two blocks?	¿Una o dos cuadras?	(oon-ah oh dohs koo-**ah**-drahs)
7.	Have you ever had surgery of the arteries in your leg?	¿Ha tenido alguna vez cirugía en las arterias de la pierna?	(ah teh-**nee**-doh ahl-**goo**-nah vehs see-roo-**hee**-ah ehn las ahr-tehr-ee-**ahs** deh lah pee-**ehr**-nah)
8.	Or an angioplasty in your leg?	¿O una angioplastia en la pierna?	(oh oon-ah ahn-hee-oh-plahs-**tee**-ah ehn lah pee-**ehr**-nah)
9.	I need to listen to the arteries in your foot with this machine	Necesito escuchar las arterias en su pie con esta máquina	(neh-seh-**see**-toh ehs-koo-**chahr** lahs ahr-tehr-**ee**-ahs ehn soo **pee**-eh kohn ehs-tah **mah**-kee-nah)
10.	It is a type of ultrasound	Es un tipo de ultrasonido	(ehs oon **tee**-poh deh ool-trah-sohn-**ee**-doh)

PHYSICAL
Section Two
EXAMINATION

1. Do this	Haga esto	(**ah**-gah **ehs**-toh)
2. I need to take your blood pressure, temperature, and pulse	Necesito tomar su presión, temperatura, y pulso	(neh-seh-**see**-toh toh-**mahr** soo preh-see-**ohn** tehm-pehr-ah-**too**-rah ee **pool**-soh)
3. Relax	Relájese	(reh-**lah**-heh-seh)
4. Sit up	Siéntese	(see-**ehn**-teh-seh)
5. Stand up	Párese	(**pah**-reh-seh)
6. Lie down	Acuéstese	(ah-koo-**ehs**-teh-seh)
7. Look here	Mire aquí	(mee-reh ah-**kee**)
8. Look there	Mire allí	(mee-reh ah-**yee**)
9. I need to listen to your heart and lungs	Necesito escuchar sus corazón y pulmones	(neh-seh-**see**-toh ehs-koo-**chahr** soos kohr-ah-**sohn** ee pool-**mohn**-ehs)
10. Breathe deeply	Respire profundamente	(reh-**spee**-reh proh-foon-doh-**mehn**-teh)
11. Hold your breath	Aguante su respiración	(ah-goo-**ahn**-teh soo rehs-peer-ah-see-**ohn**)
12. Cough	Tosa	(**toh**-sah)
13. I need to examine your abdomen	Necesito examinar su abdomen	(neh-seeh-**see**-toh ehx-ahm-ee-**nahr** soo ahb-**doh**-mehn)
14. Does it hurt here?	¿Le duele aquí?	(leh doo-**eh**-leh ah-**kee**)
15. Open your mouth	Abra la boca	(**ah**-brah lah **boh**-kah)
16. Say ahhh	Diga ahhh	(**dee**-gah ahhhh)
17. Stick out your tongue	Saqué la lengua	(sah-**keh** lah **lehn**-gwah)
18. Swallow	Trague	(**trah**-geh)
19. Turn your head to the right	Mueva su cabeza hacia la derecha	(moo-**eh**-veh soo kah-**beh**-sah ah-**see**-ah lah deh-**reh**-chah)
20. So far everything looks normal	Por ahora, todo se ve normal	(pohr ah-**ohr**-ah toh-doh seh veh nohr-**mahl**)

PATIENT
Section Three
INSTRUCTIONS

1. Take this medicine	Tome la medicina	(toh-meh lah meh-dee-**see**-nah)
2. Two times a day	Dos veces al día	(dohs **veh**-sehs ahl **dee**-ah)
3. Three times a day	Tres veces al día	(trehs **veh**-sehs ahl **dee**-ah)
4. Every 6 hours for 10 days	Cada seis horas por diez días	(kah-dah seh-ees ohr-ahs pohr dee-ehs **dee**-ahs)
5. After each meal	Después de cada comida	(dehs-**poo**-ehs deh **kah**-dah koh-**mee**-dah)
6. Breakfast, lunch, and dinner	Desayuno, almuerzo, cena	(deh-seye-**oo**-noh ahl-moo-**ehr**-soh seh-nah)
7. Each night before bedtime	Cada noche antes de acostarse	(kah-dah **noh**-cheh ahn-tehs deh ah-koh-**stahr**-seh)
8. Pills, tablets	Pastillas, tabletas	(pahs-**tee**-yahs, tah-**bleh**-tahs)
9. This is a prescription for the medicine	Esta es la receta para la medicina	(ehs-tah ehs lah reh-**seh**-tah pah-rah lah meh-dee-**see**-nah)
10. Take this prescription to the pharmacy in this hospital	Lleve esta receta a la farmacia de este hospital	(**yeh**-veh ehs-tah reh-**seh**-tah ah lah fahr-mah-**see**-ah deh ehs-teh ohs-pee-**tahl**)
11. Take this prescription to any pharmacy	Lleve esta receta a cuálquier farmacia	(**yeh**-veh ehs-tah reh-**seh**-tah ah koo-**ahl**-kee-ehr fahr-mah-**see**-ah)
12. Call me when you need more medicine	Llámeme cuándo necesite más medicinas	(**yah**-meh-meh koo-**ahn**-doh neh-seh-**see**-teh **mahs** meh-dee-**see**-nahs)
13. Ask the nurse	Consulte la enfermera	(kohn-**sool**-teh lah ehn-fehr-**mehr**-ah)
14. Ask the doctor	Consulte al doctor	(kohn-**sool**-teh ehl dohk-**tohr**)
15. Wait for the clerk	Espere por la recepcionista	(ehs-**pehr**-eh pohr lah reh-sehp-see-ohn-**ees**-tah)
16. Please wait in the waiting room	Por favor, espere en la sala de espera	(pohr-fah-**vohr** ehs-**pehr**-eh ehn lah **sah**-lah deh ehs-**pehr**-ah)

17.	You need to stay overnight in the hospital	Necesita pasar la noche en el hospital	(neh-seh-**see**-tah pah-**sahr** lah **noh**-cheh ehn ehl ohs-pee-**tahl**)
18.	You will be admitted	Lo vamos a internar en el hospital	(loh **vah**-mohs ah een-tehr-**nahr** ehn ehl ohs-pee-**tahl**)
19.	You will be discharged today	Lo vamos a dar de alta hoy	(loh **vah**-mohs ah dahr deh **ahl**-tah oy)
20.	You can go home today in the afternoon	Puede irse a su casa hoy por la tarde	(poo-**eh**-deh **eer**-seh ah soo **kah**-sah oy pohr lah **tahr**-deh)
21.	You can go home tomorrow	Puede irse a su casa mañana	(poo-**eh**-deh **eer**-seh ah soo **kah**-sah ma-**nyah**-nah)
22.	Return to the clinic in two weeks	Regrese a la clínica en dos semanas	(reh-**greh**-seh ah lah **klee**-nee-kah en dohs seh-**mehn**-ahs)
23.	Call or return to the ER if these symptoms occur	Llame o regrese a la sala de emergencia si estos síntomás occuren	(**yah**-meh oh reh-**greh**-seh ah lah **sah**-lah deh eh-mehr-hehn-**see**-ah see ehs-tohs **seen**-toh-mahs oh-koo-**rehn**)
24.	Increasing pain	Aumento del dolor	(ah-oo-**mehn**-toh dehl doh-**lohr**)
25.	Increased bleeding	Aumento del sangramiento	(ah-oo-**mehn**-toh dehl sahn-grah-mee-**ehn**-toh)
26.	Excessive sleepiness	Sueño excesivo	(soo-**eh**-nyoh ehx-seh-**see**-voh)
27.	Numbness in your fingers	Los dedos de las manos o los pies adormecidos	(los **deh**-dohs deh lahs **mah**-nohs oh los **pee**-ehs ah-dohr-meh-**see**-dohs)
28.	Fever	Fiebre	(fee-**eh**-breh)
29.	Increased shortness of breath	Aumenta la dificultad al respirar	(ah-oo-**mehn**-tah la dee-fee-kool-**tahd** ahl reh-speer-**ahr**)
30.	Here is the phone number	Aquí está el número de teléfono	(ah-**kee** ehs-**tah** ehl **noo**-mehr-oh deh teh-**leh**-foh-noh)

Section Four

LABORATORY TESTS

1. What test are you here for?	¿Qué prueba va a tener?	(**keh** proo-**eh**-bah vah ah teh-**neer**)
2. Do you have a note from your doctor?	¿Tiene una nota de su doctor?	(tee-**ehn**-eh oon-ah **noh**-tah deh soo dohk-**tohr**)
3. Did you eat breakfast?	¿Tomó desayuno?	(toh-**moh** deh-seye-**oo**-noh)
4. You need a blood test	Necesita una prueba de sangre	(neh-seh-**see**-tah oon-ah proo-**eh**-bah deh **sahn**-greh)
5. Make a fist	Haga un puño	(**ah**-gah oon poo-**nyoh**)
6. You will feel a little stick	Sentirá un pinchazo	(sehn-tee-**rah** oon peen-**chah**-soh)
7. Apply pressure here for 5 minutes	Aplique presión por cinco minutos	(ah-plee-keh preh-see-**ohn** pohr **seen**-koh mee-**noo**-tohs)
8. Do you want a bandaid?	¿Quiere un vendaje?	(kee-**ehr**-eh oon vehn-**dah**-heh)
9. Your sugar level is high	Su nivel de azúcar está alto	(soo nee-**vehl** deh ah-**soo**-kahr ehs-**tah** ahl-toh)
10. You may have diabetes	Es posible que usted tenga díabetes	(ehs poh-**see**-bleh keh oos-**tehd** tehn-gah **dee**-ah-beh-tehs)
11. You need another sugar test	Necesita otra prueba de azúcar	(neh-seh-**see**-tah oh-trah proo-**eh**-bah deh ah-**soo**-kahr)
12. Your creatinine level is high	Su nivel de creatinina está alto	(soo nee-**vehl** deh kreh-ah-tee-**nee**-nah ehs-**tah** ahl-toh)
13. This indicates a problem with the kidneys	Usualmente esto indica un problema con sus riñones	(oo-soo-ahl-**mehn**-teh ehs-toh een-**dee**-kah oon proh-**bleh**-mah kohn lohs ree-**nyohn**-ehs)
14. Your white blood cell count is high	Los glóbulos blancos están altos	(lohs **gloh**-boo-lohs **blahn**-kohs ehs-**tahn** ahl-tohs)
15. You probably have an infection	Probablamente tiene un infección	(proh-bah-blah-**mehn**-teh tee-**eh**-neh oon eeh-fehk-see-**ohn**)
16. You need to have blood cultures	Necesita cultivos de la sangre	(neh-seh-**see**-tah kool-**tee**-vohs deh lah **sahn**-greh)

17.	The purpose of these tests is to check for AIDS and hepatitis	El propósito de esta prueba es para chequear la SIDA y hepatitis	(ehl proh-**poh**-see-toh deh ehs-tah proo-**eh**-bah ehs pah-rah cheh-**keh**-ahr lah **see**-dah ee eh-pah-**tee**-tees)
18.	Your tests of coagulation are abnormal	Su prueba de coagulación es anormal	(soo proo-**eh**-bah deh koh-ah-goo-lah-see-**ohn** ehs ah-nohr-**mahl**)
19.	We will need to postpone the procedure for at least one day	Necesitaremos posponer el procedimiento por lo menos un día más	(neh-seh-see-tahr-**eh**-mohs pohst-pohn-**ehr** ehl proh-seh-dee-mee-**ehn**-toh pohr loh **meh**-nohs oon **dee**-ah **mahs**)
20.	Sodium	Sodio	(soh-**dee**-oh)
21.	Potassium	Potasio	(poh-tah-**see**-oh)
22.	Cholesterol	Colesterol	(koh-lehs-tehr-**ohl**)
23.	You have anemia	Tiene anemia	(tee-**ehn**-eh ah-neh-**mee**-ah)
24.	Red blood cells transport oxygen from the lungs to all of the body	Los glóbulos rojos transportan oxígeno de los pulmones al resto del cuerpo	(lohs **gloh**-boo-lohs roh-hohs trahns-pohr-tahn ohx-**ee**-heh-noh deh lohs pool-mohn-ehs ahl rehs-toh dehl koo-ehr-poh)
25.	You need a urine test	Necesita una prueba de orina	(neh-seh-**see**-tah oon-ah proo-**eh**-bah deh oh-**ree**-nah)
26.	Go to the bathroom	Vaya a ese baño	(veye-ah ah eh-seh **bah**-nyoh)
27.	After urinating a little bit in the toilet	Después de orinar un poco en el inodoro	(dehs-poo-**ehs** deh oh-ree-**nahr** oon poh-koh ehn ehl een-oh-**dohr**-oh)
28.	Put the rest into this cup and return here	Ponga el resto en este recipiente y regrese aquí	(**pohn**-gah ehl **rehs**-toh ehn ehs-teh reh-see-pee-**ehn**-teh ee reh-**greh**-seh ah-**kee**)
29.	You can call tomorrow for the results	Puede llamar mañana por los resultados	(poo-**eh**-deh yah-**mahr** mah-**nyah**-nah pohr lohs reh-sool-**tah**-dohs)

30.	Here is the phone number	Aquí esta el número de teléfono	(ah-**kee** ehs-**tah** ehl **noo**-mehr-oh deh teh-**leh**-foh-noh)
31.	Your doctor will discuss the results with you	Su doctor discutirá los resultados con usted	(soo dohk-**tohr** dees-koo-teer-**ah** lohs reh-sool-**tah**-dohs kohn oos-**tehd**)

PROCEDURES

Section Five

1. ARTERIAL BLOOD GAS

1. The purpose of this test is to check the exact oxygen level in your blood	El propósito de esta prueba es chequear la cantidad exacta de oxígeno en la sangre	(ehl proh-**poh**-see-toh deh ehs-tah proo-**eh**-bah ehs chech-keh-**ahr** lah kahn-tee-**dahd** ehx-**ahk**-tah deh ohx-**ee**-heh-noh ehn lah **sahn**-greh)
2. Make a fist	Haga un puño	(**ah**-gah oon poo-**nyoh**)
3. Open your hand	Abra la mano	(**ah**-breh lah **mah**-noh)
4. You will feel a little stick	Sentirá un pinchazo	(sehn-teer-**ah** oon peen-**chah**-soh)

2. BRONCHOSCOPY

1. The purpose of this test is to check for cancer	El propósito de esta prueba es chequear la posibilidad de cancer	(ehl proh-**poh**-see-toh deh ehs-tah proo-**eh**-bah ehs cheh-keh-**ahr** lah poh-see-beel-ee-**dahd** deh **kahn**-sehr)
2. We will need to do a biopsy	Necesitaremos hacer una biopsia	(neh-seh-see-tahr-**eh**-mohs ah-**sehr** oon-ah bee-op-**see**-ah)
3. The tube will go through your mouth and then down to your lungs	El tubo irá por su boca y después hacia el pulmón	(ehl too-boh ee-**rah** pohr soo **boh**-kah ee dehs-poo-**ehs** ah-**see**-ah ehl pool-**mohn**)
4. The risks include collapse of the lung	Los riesgos incluyen la caída del pulmon	(lohs ree-**ehs**-gohs een-kloo-**yehn** lah kah-**ee**-dah dehl pool-**mohn**)

5. Bleeding	Hemorragia	(eh-mohr-ah-**hee**-ah)
6. Increased shortness of breath	Aumento de la dificultad al respirar	(ah-oo-**mehn**-toh deh lah dee-fee-kool-**tahd** ahl rehs-peer-**ahr**)
7. Which will prevent us from completing the procedure	Lo cuál nos prevenirá para completar el procedimiento	(loh koo-**ahl** nohs preh-veh-neer-**ah** pah-rah kohm-pleh-**tahr** ehl proh-seh-dee-mee-**ehn**-toh)
8. It is also possible that the biopsy will not give us the diagnosis	También, es posible que la biopsia no nos dé el diagnóstico	(tahm-bee-**ehn** ehs poh-**see**-bleh keh lah bee-ohp-**see**-ah noh nohs **deh** ehl dee-ahg-**nohs**-tee-koh)
9. Do you understand?	¿Entiende?	(ehn-tee-**ehn**-deh)

3. CENTRAL VENOUS CATHETERIZATION

1. Your doctor has asked us to place an IV in your neck	Su doctor solicitó una línea intravenosa en su cuello	(soo dohk-**tohr** soh-lee-see-**toh** oon-ah **lee**-neh-ah een-trah-vehn-**oh**-sah ehn soo koo-**eh**-yoh)
2. It allows us to feed you through your veins	Nos ayuda a darle comida líquida a través de las venas	(nohs eye-oo-dah ah **dahr**-leh koh-**mee**-dah **lee**-kee-dah ah trah-**vehs** deh lahs **veh**-nahs)
3. Until your intestines are working better	Hasta que sus intestinos comienzen a trabajar mejor	(ah-stah keh soos een-tehs-**tee**-nohs koh-mee-ehn-**sehn** ah trah-bah-**hahr** meh-**hohr**)
4. The risks include collapse of the lung	Los riesgos incluyen la caída del pulmón	(lohs ree-ehs-gohs een-kloo-yehn lah kah-**ee**-dah dehl pool-**mohn**)

5. Injury to the artery with bleeding and formation of a hematoma	Daño a la arteria con hemorragia y la formación de hematoma	(dah-nyoh ah lah ahr-tehr-ee-ah kohn eh-mohr-ah-hee-ah ee lah fohr-mah-see-**ohn** deh eh-mah-toh-mah)
6. Malposition	Malposición	(mahl-poh-see-see-**ohn**)
7. Sometimes the catheter does not go to the correct position	A veces el catéter no va a la posición correcta	(ah veh-sehs ehl kah-**teh**-tehr noh vah ah lah poh-see-see-**ohn** kohr-ehk-tah)
8. And we need to reposition it	Y necesitamos reponerlo	(ee neh-seh-see-**tah**-mohs reh-pohn-**ehr**-loh)
9. The alternative is to use ultrasound guidance	La alternativa es guiar la aguja y catéter con ultrasonido	(lah ahl-tehr-nah-**tee**-vah ehs goo-ee-**ahr** lah ah-**goo**-hah ee kah-**teh**-tehr kohn ool-trah-sohn-**ee**-doh)
10. This takes longer, but it is safer	Se tarda más pero es más seguro	(seh tahr-dah **mahs** peh-roh ehs **mahs** seh-goo-roh)

4. CHEST TUBE PLACEMENT

1. The purpose of this procedure is	El propósito de este procedimiento	(ehl proh-**poh**-see-toh deh ehs-teh proh-seh-dee-mee-**ehn**-toh)
2. To remove the air or fluid from around your lungs	Es remover el aire o fluído alrededor de sus pulmones	(ehs reh-moh-**vehr** ehl ah-**ee**-reh oh floo-**ee**-doh ahl-reh-deh-**dohr** deh soos pool-**mohn**-ehs)
3. We will give you local anesthesia	Le daremos anestesia local	(leh dahr-**eh**-mohs ahn-ehs-tehs-**ee**-ah loh-**kahl**)
4. However, we are unable to completely prevent pain	Sin embargo no podemos evitar el dolor completamente	(seen ehm-**bahr**-goh noh poh-**deh**-mohs eh-vee-**tahr** ehl doh-**lohr** kohm-pleh-tah-**mehn**-teh)

5. After the tube is in position	Después qué el tubo esta en posición	(dehs-poo-**ehs** keh ehl **too**-boh ehs-tah ehn poh-see-see-**ohn**)
6. You will be able to take pain medicines by mouth	Puede tomar medicinas para el dolor por la boca	(poo-**eh**-deh toh-**mahr** meh-dee-**see**-nahs pah-rah ehl doh-**lohr** pohr lah **boh**-kah)
7. Usually the tube stays in for 1 to 4 days	Usualmente, el tubo se queda adentro por uno a cuatro días	(oos-oo-ahl-**mehn**-teh ehl too-boh seh **kweh**-dah ah-**dehn**-troh pohr oon-oh ah koo-**ahn**-troh **dee**-ahs)

5. COLONOSCOPY

1. The purpose of this test is to check for cancer or other causes of bleeding	El propósito de este prueba es chequear cáncer y otras causas de hemorragia	(ehl proh-**poh**-see-toh deh ehs-teh proo-**eh**-bah ehs cheh-keh-**ahr kahn**-sehr ee oh-trohs kah-oo-sahs deh ehm-ohr-ah-**hee**-ah)
2. It is important that you follow the instructions	Es importante que usted siga las instrucciones	(ehs eem-pohr-**tahn**-teh keh oos-**tehd** see-gah lahs een-strook-see-**ohn**-ehs)
3. And take the diet of liquids and the laxative the night before	Y tome los líquidos y el laxante la noche anterior	(ee toh-meh lohs **lee**-kee-dohs ee ehl lahx-**ahn**-teh lah **noh**-che ahn-tehr-ee-**ohr**)
4. You will be given medicine to help decrease your discomfort	Le daremos medicina para disminuir su molestia	(leh dahr-**eh**-mohs meh-dee-**see**-nah pah-rah dees-mee-noo-**eer** soo moh-lehs-**tee**-ah)
5. The procedure takes about one hour	El procedimeinto tarda cerca de una hora	(ehl proh-seh-dee-mee-**ehn**-toh tahr-dah **sehr**-kah deh oon-ah **ohr**-ah)

6. ELECTROCARDIOGRAM

1. The purpose of this test is to check the rhythm of the heart	El propósito de esta prueba es chequear el ritmo del corazón	(ehl proh-**poh**-see-toh deh ehs-tah proo-**eh**-bah ehs cheh-keh-**ahr** ehl **reet**-moh dehl kohr-ah-**sohn**)
2. Is is also helpful to check ischemia and myocardial infarction	También ayuda a chequear la isquemia e infarto cardíaco	(tahm-bee-**ehn** eye-oo-dah ah cheh-keh-**ahr** lah ees-keh-**mee**-ah ee een-**fahr**-toh kahr-**dee**-ahk-oh)
3. Heart attack	Ataque al corazón	(ah-tah-keh ahl kohr-ah-**sohn**)
4. It does not hurt	No le duele	(noh leh doo-**ehl**-eh)
5. It is important that you do not move while the machine is on	Es importante que no se mueva cuando la máquina está funcionando	(ehs eem-pohr-**tahn**-teh keh noh seh moo-**eh**-vah koo-**ahn**-doh lah **mah**-kee-nah ehs-**tah** foon-see-ohn-**ahn**-doh)

7. HEEL STICK

1. The purpose of this test is to obtain a small sample of blood	El propósito de este prueba es obtener una muestra pequeña de sangre	(ehl proh-**poh**-see-toh deh ehs-teh proo-**eh**-bah ehs ohb-teh-**nehr** oon-ah moo-**ehs**-trah peh-keh-**nyah** deh **sahn**-greh)
2. Which will be sent to the laboratory	Que se enviará al laboratorio	(keh seh ehn-vee-ahr-**ah** ahl lah-bohr-oh-tohr-**ee**-oh)

3. Only a few drops of blood	Solamente unas gotas de sangre	(soh-lah-**mehn**-teh oon-ahs **goh**-tahs deh **sahn**-greh)
4. Are removed from the heel of the baby	Se sacarán del talón del bebé	(seh sah-kahr-**ahn** dehl tah-**lohn** dehl beh-**beh**)

8. INTRAVENOUS LINE PLACEMENT

1. I need to start an IV	Necesito comenzar una línea intravenosa	(neh-seh-**see**-toh koh-mehn-**sahr** oon-ah **lee**-neh-ah een-trah-vehn-**oh**-sah)
2. Make a fist	Haga un puño	(**ah**-ga oon poo-**nyoh**)
3. You will feel a little stick	Sentirá un pinchazo	(sehn-teer-**ah** oon peen-**chah**-soh)

9. LUMBAR PUNCTURE

1. The purpose of this test is to check for meningitis	El propósito de esta prueba es chequear meningitis	(ehl proh-**poh**-see-toh deh ehs-tah proo-**eh**-bah ehs cheh-keh-**ahr** meh-neen-**hee**-tees)
2. A small needle will be put into the sac of fluid which surrounds the spinal cord	Una aguja pequeña se pondrá en el saco de fluído alrededor de la médula espinal	(oon-ah ah-goo-hah peh-keh-**nyah** seh pohn-**drah** ehn ehl **sah**-koh deh floo-**ee**-doh ahl-reh-deh-**dohr** deh lah **meh**-doo-lah ehs-pee-**nahl**)
3. A small amount of fluid will be removed	Se le sacará una cantidad pequeña de fluído	(seh leh sah-kah-**rah** oon-ah kahn-tee-**dahd** peh-keh-**nyah** deh floo-**ee**-doh)

4. This procedure has a risk of causing an infection	Este procedimiento tiene un riesgo de causar una infección	(ehs-teh pro-seh-dee-mee-**ehn**-toh tee-**ehn**-eh oon ree-**ehs**-goh deh kah-oo-**sahr** oon-ah een-fehk-see-**ohn**)
5. However, this is very uncommon	Sin embargo, no es común	(seen ehm-**bahr**-goh noh ehs koh-**moon**)
6. The most common side effect is a headache	El problema más común es dolor de cabeza	(ehl proh-**bleh**-mah **mahs** koh-**moon** ehs doh-**lohr** deh kah-**beh**-sah)
7. To help prevent this	Para ayudar a evitar esto	(pah-rah eye-oo-**dahr** ah eh-vee-**tahr** ehs-toh)
8. You will need to stay flat on your back in bed for the rest of the day	Nesesitará quedarse boca arriba en la cama el resto del día	(neh-seh-see-tahr-**ah** keh-**dahr**-seh boh-kah ah-**ree**-bah ehn lah **cah**-mah ehl **rehs**-toh dehl **dee**-ah)
9. However, you may elevate your head with one or two pillows	Sin embargo, puede elevar su cabeza con una o dos almohadas	(seen ehm-**bahr**-goh poo-**eh**-deh eh-leh-**vahr** soo kah-**beh**-sah kohn oon-ah o dohs ahl-moh-**ah**-dahs)
10. It is also good to drink a lot of liquids	También, es bueno tomar muchos líquidos	(tahm-bee-**ehn** ehs boo-**eh**-noh toh-**mahr** **moo**-chohs **lee**-kee-dohs)

10. NASOGASTRIC TUBE PLACEMENT

1. The purpose of this procedure is to check for blood in your stomach or help decompress your intestines	El propósito de esta prueba es para chequear si hay sangre en el estómago o ayudar a descomprimir sus intestinos	(ehl proh-**poh**-see-toh deh ehs-tah proh-seh-dee-mee-**ehn**-toh ehs pah-rah cheh-keh-**ahr** see eye **sahn**-greh ehn ehl ehs-**toh**-mah-goh oh eye-oo-**dahr** ah dehs-kohm-pree-**meer** soos een-tehs-**tee**-nohs)

2. Sit up	Siéntese	(see-**ehn**-tee-seh)
3. Take a sip of water	Tome un poco de agua	(toh-meh oon **poh**-koh deh ah-gwah)
4. Swallow	Trague	(**trah**-geh)
5. Do not touch the tube	No toque el tubo	(noh **toh**-keh ehl **too**-boh)

11. PARACENTESIS

1. The purpose of this procedure	El propósito de este procedimiento	(ehl proh-**poh**-see-toh deh ehs-teh proh-seh-dee-mee-**ehn**-toh)
2. Is to remove fluid from the abdomen	Es para extraer fluído del abdomen	(ehs pah-rah ehx-trah-**ehr** floo-**ee**-doh dehl ahb-**doh**-mehn)
3. To check for infection or cancer	Y para chequear por infección o cáncer	(ee pah-rah cheh-keh-**ahr** pohr een-fehk-see-**ohn** oh **kahn**-sehr)
4. And to help you breathe more easily	Y para ayudarle a respirar más fácilmente	(ee pah-rah eye-oo-**dahr**-leh ah reh-speer-**ahr** mahs fah-seel-**mehn**-teh)
5. The main risk is that the needle could hit the intestine and cause an infection	El mayor riesgo es que la aguja podría tocar el intestino y causar una infección	(ehl mah-**yohr** ree-**ehs**-goh ehs keh lah ah-**goo**-hah poh-**dree**-ah toh-kahr ehl een-tehs-**tee**-noh ee ksh-oo-**sahr** oon-ah een-fehk-see-**ohn**)
6. However, this is very uncommon	Sin embargo, esto es muy raro	(seen ehm-**bahr**-goh ehs-toh ehs moy **rahr**-oh)
7. We will use U/S to guide the needle and help avoid the bowel	Usaremos ultrasonido para guiar la aguja y evitar dañar el intestino	(oos-ahr-**eh**-mohs ool-trah-soh-**nee**-doh pah-rah goo-ee-**ahr** lah ah-**goo**-hah ee eh-vee-**tahr** dah-**nyahr** ehl een-tehs-**tee**-noh)

12. PERITONEAL LAVAGE

1. The purpose of this test is to check for internal bleeding	El próposito de esta prueba es chequear si hay hemorragia interna	(ehl **proh**-poh-see-toh deh ehs-tah proo-**eh**-bah ehs cheh-keh-**ahr** see eye ehm-ohr-ah-**hee**-ah een-**tehr**-nah)
2. A catheter is placed into the abdomen	Un catéter coloca en el abdomen	(oon kah-**teh**-tehr koh-**loh**-kah ehn ehl ahb-**doh**-mehn)
3. And about 1 liter of fluid is put into the abdominal cavity	Y un litro de fluído es introducido dentro del abdomen	(ee oon **lee**-troh deh floo-**ee**-doh ehs een-troh-doo-**see**-doh dehn-troh dehl ahb-**doh**-mehn)
4. The fluid is then removed	Entonces, se extrae fluído	(ehn-**tohn**-sehs, seh ehks-**trah**-eh floo-**ee**-doh)
5. And examined for blood and other abnormalities	Y se examina para ver si hay sangre	(ee seh ehx-ah-**mee**-nah pah-rah vehr see eye **sahn**-greh)
6. The risks of this procedure are	Los riesgos de este procedimiento son	(lohs ree-**ehs**-gohs deh ehs-teh proh-seh-dee-mee-**ehn**-toh sohn)
7. Infection, bleeding and injury to the bowel	Infección, hemorragia y daño al intestino	(een-fehk-see-**ohn** ehm-ohr-ah-**hee**-ah ee dah-nyoh ahl een-tehs-**tee**-noh)

13. SKIN TEST

1. The purpose of this test is to check for exposure to TB	El propósito de este prueba es ver si ha estado expuesto a la tuberculosis	(ehl proh-**poh**-see-toh deh ehs-tah proo-**eh**-bah ehs vehr see ah ehs-**tah**-doh ehx-poo-**ehs**-toh ah lah too-behr-koo-**loh**-sees)

2. Return to the clinic in 2 days	Regrese a la clínica en dos días	(reh-**greh**-seh ah la **klee**-nee-kah en dohs **dee**-ahs)
3. And we will check the result	Y chequearemos el resultado	(ee cheh-keh-ahr-**eh**-mohs ehl reh-sool-**tah**-doh)

14. THORACENTESIS

1. The purpose of this procedure	El propósito de este procedimiento	(ehl proh-**poh**-see-toh deh ehs-teh proh-seh-dee-mee-**ehn**-toh)
2. Is to remove fluid from the space around the lungs	Es extraer fluído del espacio alrededor de los pulmones	(ehs ehks-trah-**ehr** floo-**ee**-doh dehl ehs-pah-**see**-oh ahl-reh-deh-**dohr** deh los pool-**mohn**-ehs)
3. The fluid will be sent to the laboratory to check for infection or cancer	El fluído se enviará al laboratorio para chequear infección o cáncer	(ehl floo-**ee**-doh seh ehn-vee-ah-**rah** ahl lah-bohr-ah-tohr-ee-oh pah-rah cheh-keh-ahr een-fehk-see-**ohn** oh **kahn**-sehr)
4. Hopefully this will help you to breathe more easily and better	Espero, esto le ayude a respirar más facilmente y mejor	(ehs-**pehr**-oh ehs-toh leh eye-**co**-deh ah rehs-pehr-**ahr mahs** fah-seel-**mehn**-teh ee meh-**hohr**)
5. I will give you a local anesthetic	Le daré anestesia local	(leh dahr-**eh** ahn-ehs-tehs-**ee**-ah loh-**kahl**)
6. Then a small needle will be put into one pleural space	Entonces le pondremos una aguja dentro del espacio pleural	(ehn-**tohn**-sehs leh pohn-**dreh**-mohs oon-ah ah-**goo**-hah dehn-troh dehl ehs-pah-**see**-oh pleh-oo-**rahl**)
7. After the procedure you will have a CXR	Después del procedimiento tendrá una radiografía del pecho	(dehs-poo-**ehs** dehl proh-seh-dee-mee-**ehn**-toh tehn-**drah** oon-ah rah-dee-oh-grah-**fee**-ah dehl **peh**-choh)

8. If there is abnormal air in the space around the lung	Si hay aire anormal en el espacio alrededor del pulmón	(see eye ah-**ee**-reh ah-nohr-**mahl** ehn ehl eh-spah-**see**-oh ahl-reh-deh-**dohr** dehl pool-**mohn**)
9. You will need a second CXR one hour later	Necesitará una segunda radiografía una hora más tarde	(neh-seh-see-tahr-**ah** oon-ah seh-**goon**-dah rah-dee-oh-grah-**fee**-ah oon-ah ohr-ah **mahs** tahr-deh)
10. If the lung has collapsed or you are short of breath	Si el pulmón se ha caído o tiene dificultad al respirar	(see ehl pool-**mohn** eh ah kah-**ee**-doh oh tee-**ehn**-eh dee-fee-kool-**tahd** ahl reh-speer-**ahr**)
11. You will need a chest tube	Necesitará un tubo en el pecho	(neh-seh-see-tahr-**ah** oon too-boh ehn ehl **peh**-choh)
12. This could keep you in the hospital for 1 to 3 days	Es posible que usted necesite quedarse en el hospital de uno a tres días	(ehs poh-**see**-bleh keh oos-tehd neh-seh-**see**-teh keh-**dahr**-seh ehn ehl ohs-pee-**tahl** deh oon-oh ah trehs **dee**-ahs)

15. URINARY BLADDER CATHETERIZATION

1. The purpose of this procedure is to monitor the function of the kidneys	El propósito de este procedimiento es monitorear la función de los riñones	(ehl proh-**poh**-see-toh deh ehs-teh proh-seh-dee-mee-**ehn**-toh ehs mohn-ee-tohr-ee-**ahr** lah foon-see-**ohn** deh lohs ree-**nyoh**-nehs)
2. Or to decompress the bladder	O descomprimir la vejiga	(oh dehs-kohm-pree-**meer** lah veh-**hee**-gah)
3. Lie down on your back	Acuéstese sobre su espalda	(ah-koo-**ehs**-teh-seh soh-breh soo ehs-**pahl**-dah)

4. Put your heels together	Ponga sus talones juntos	(pohn-gah soos tah-**lohn**-ehs **hoon**-tohs)
5. We will remove the catheter tomorrow	Sacaremos el catéter mañana	(sah-kahr-**eh**-mohs ehl kah-**teh**-tehr man-**nyah**-nah)

IMAGING
Section Six
STUDIES

1. BARIUM STUDIES

COOKIE SWALLOW

1.	The purpose of this test is to check your ability to swallow	El propósito de esta prueba es chequear su habilidad de tragar	(ehl proh-**poh**-see-toh deh ehs-tah proo-**eh**-bah ehs cheh-keh-**arh** soo ah-beel-ee-**dahd** deh trah-**gahr**)
2.	And to prevent food from going into your airway	Y evitar que la comida se vaya por la tráquea	(ee eh-vee-**tahr** keh lah koh-**mee**-dah seh veye-ah pohr lah **trah**-keh-ah)
3.	Sit here	Siéntese aquí	(see-**ehn**-teh-seh ah-**kee**)
4.	Take a sip/drink and hold/keep it in your mouth	Tome un trago y manténgalo en su boca	(toh-meh oon **trah**-goh ee mahn-**tehn**-gah-loh ehn soo **boh**-kah)
5.	Hold this	Aguante esto	(ah-goo-**ahn**-teh ehs-toh)
6.	Drink	Tome	(**toh**-meh)
7.	Swallow	Trague	(**trah**-geh)
8.	Chew this cracker and hold/keep it in your mouth	Mastique esta galleta y manténgala en su boca	(mahs-tee-keh ehs-tah gah-**yeh**-tah ee mahn-**tehn**-gah-lah ehn soo boh-kah)
9.	You need to drink more	Necesita tomar más	(neh-seh-**see**-tah toh-mahr **mahs**)

UGI

1.	The purpose of this test is to examine your esophagus, stomach and duodenum	El propósito de esta prueba es examinar el esófago, estómago y duodeno	(Ehl pro-**poh**-see-toh deh ehs-tah proo-**eh**-bah ehs ehx-ahm-een-**ahr** ehl eh-**soh**-fah-goh eh-**stohm**-ah-goh ee doo-oh-**dehn**-oh)

2. Did you eat breakfast?	¿Tomó desayuno?	(toh-**moh** deh-seye-oon-oh)
3. You will drink barium (a white liquid)	Tomará bario, un líquido blanco	(toh-mahr-**ah** bahr-ee-oh oon **lee**-kee-doh blahn-koh)
4. And we will take x-rays	Y le tomaremos radiografías	(ee leh toh-mahr-**eh**-mohs rah-dee-oh-grah-**fee**-ahs)
5. Stand here	Párese aquí	(**pahr**-rh-seh ah-**kee**)
6. Turn a little bit to the left	Muévase un poco hacia la izquierda	(moo-**eh**-vah-se oon poh-koh ah-**see**-ah lah ees-kee-**ehr**-dah)
7. Swallow these crystals	Trague este polvo	(**trah**-geh ehs-teh **pohl**-voh)
8. Drink this water	Tome esta agua	(toh-meh ehs-tah ah-**goo**-ah)
9. Do not burp	No eructe	(noh eh-**rook**-teh)
10. Do not drink the barium until I tell you	No se tome el bario hasta que yo le diga	(noh seh toh-meh ehl bahr-**ee**-oh ahs-tah keh yoh leh **dee**-gah)
11. Drink	Tome	(**toh**-meh)
12. The table will now go down	Ahora la mesa va hacia abajo	(ah-ohr-ah lah **meh**-sah vah aha-see-ah ah-**bah**-hoh)
13. Turn on your left side	Virese a su lado izquierdo	(veer-**eh**-seh ah soo lah-doh ees-kee-**ehr**-doh)
14. Turn more	Virese más	(veer-eh-seh **mahs**)
15. Drink through this straw	Tome con este pajita	(**toh**-meh kohn ehs-teh pah-**hee**-tah)
16. The table will now go up	Ahora la mesa va hacia arriba	(ah-**ohr**-ah lah **meh**-sah vah ah-**see**-ah ah-**ree**-bah)
17. Do you feel the platform under your feet?	¿Siente la plataforma debajo de sus pies?	(see-**ehn**-teh lah plah-tah-**fohr**-mah deh-**bah**-hoh deh soos pee-**ehs**)
18. We are almost finished	Casi terminamos	(kah-see tehr-mee-**nah**-mohs)

19.	We need a few more pictures	Necesitamos unas cuantas más radiografías	(neh-seh-see-**tah**-mohs oon-ahs koo-**ahn**-tahs **mahs** rah-dee-oh-grah-**fee**-ahs)
20.	That is all	Eso es todo	(**ehs**-oh ehs **toh**-doh)
21.	You should drink a lot of water today to help avoid constipation	Debe tomar mucha agua hoy para evitar constipación	(**deh**-beh toh-**mahr** moo-choh ah-**goo**-ah oy pah-rah ay-vee-**tahr** kohn-stee-pah-see-**ohn**)

SMALL BOWEL FOLLOW THROUGH

1.	The purpose of this test	El propósito de esta prueba	(ehl proh-**poh**-see-toh deh ehs-tah proo-**eh**-bah)
2.	Is to check for obstruction or other abnormalities in the small bowel	Es chequear la obstrucción u otras anormalidades del intestino delgado	(ehs cheh-keh-**ahr** lah ohbs-trook-see-**ohn** oo oh-trahs ah-nohr-mahl-ee-**dah**-dehs dehl een-tehs-**teen**-oh dehl-**gah**-doh)
3.	You will need to drink several cups of barium	Necesita tomar varios vasos de bario	(neh-seh-**see**-tah toh-**mahr** vahr-**ee**-ahs **vah**-sohs deh bahr-**ee**-oh)
4.	Then we will take x-rays	Entonces tomaremos las radiografías	(ehn-**tohn**-sehs toh-mahr-**eh**-mohs lahs rah-dee-oh-grah-**fee**-ahs)

LGI

1.	The purpose of this test	El propósito de esta prueba	(ehl proh-**poh**-see-toh de ehs-tah proo-**eh**-bah)
2.	Is to check for cancer or polyps in the large bowel	Es chequear cáncer o pólipos en el intestino grueso	(ehs cheh-keh-**ahr** **kahn**-sehr oh **poh**-lee-pohs ehn ehl een-tehs-**teen**-oh groo-**eh**-soh)
3.	Did you take the laxative last night?	¿Tomó el laxante anoche?	(toh-**moh** ehl lahx-**ahn**-teh ah-**noh**-cheh)

4. The barium is going in	El bario está entrando	(ehl bahr-**ee**-oh ehs-**tah** ehn-**trahn**-doh)
5. Take deep slow breaths	Respire profundo y despacio	(reh-**spee**-reh proh-**foon**-doh ee dehs-**pah**-see-oh)
6. The air is now going in	El aire está entrando	(ehl ah-**ee**-reh ehs-**tah** ehn-**trahn**-doh)
7. Are you o.k.?	¿Está bien?	(ehs-**tah** bee-**ehn**)
8. Turn on your left side	Virese a la izquierda	(vee-**reh**-seh ah lah ees-kee-**ehr**-dah)
9. Turn on your stomach	Virese boca abajo	(vee-**reh**-seh boh-kah ah-**bah**-hoh)
10. Turn on your back	Virese boca arriba	(vee-**reh**-seh boh-kah ah-**ree**-bah)

2. COMPUTED TOMOGRAPHY

1. You are here for a CT scan	Usted esta aquí para una tomografía computarizada	(oos-tehd ehs-tah ah-**kee** pah-rah oon-ah toh-moh-grah-**fee**-ah kohm-poo-tahr-ee-sah-dah)
2. Did you drink the barium last night?	¿Tomó el bario anoche?	(toh-**moh** ehl bahr-ee-oh ah-**noh**-cheh)
3. Are you allergic to contrast or iodine?	¿Es usted alérgico a la tinta de radiografías?	(ehs oos-tehd ah-**lehr**-hee-koh ah lah teen-tah deh rah-dee-oh-grah-**fee**-ahs)
4. Have you ever had a CT scan or angiogram?	¿Ha tenido algúna vez una tomografía computarizada o angiograma?	(ah teh-**nee**-doh ahl-**goon**-ah vehs oon-ah toh-moh-grah-**fee**-ah kohm-poo-tahr-ee-**sah**-dah oh ahn-hee-oh-**grah**-mah)

5. Did you have any problems with the contrast?	¿Tuvo algún problema con la tinta?	(too-voh ahl-**goon** proh-**bleh**-mah kohn lah **teen**-tah)
6. Did you have shortness of breath?	¿Tiene dificultad al respirar?	(tee-**ehn**-eh dee-fee-kool-**tahd** ahl reh-speer-**ahr**)
7. Rash?	¿Erupción?	(ehr-oop-see-**ohn**)
8. Itching?	¿Picazón?	(pee-kah-**sohn**)
9. Vomiting?	¿Vómitos?	(**voh**-mee-tohs)
10. Did the doctor give you any medicine?	¿Le dió el doctor alguna medicina?	(lah **dee**-oh ehl dohk-**tohr** ahl-**goon**-ah meh-dee-**see**-nah)
11. This test takes about 15 minutes	Esta prueba se tarda quince minutos	(ehs-tah proo-**eh**-bah seh **tahr**-dah keen-seh mee-**noh**-tohs)
12. You need to have an IV	Necesita una línea intravenosa	(neh-seh-**see**-tah oon-ah **leen**-eh-ah een-trah-vehn-**oh**-sah)
13. The contrast is going in	La tinta está entrando	(lah teen-tah ehs-**tah** ehn-**trahn**-doh)
14. Does your arm feel o.k.?	¿Siente su brazo bien?	(see-**ehn**-teh soo **brah**-soh bee-**ehn**)
15. Call us if your arm starts to hurt or becomes swollen	Llámenos si su brazo le duele o nota hinchazón	(**yah**-meh-nohs see so **brah**-soh leh doo-**eh**-leh oh noh-tah een-chah-**sohn**)
16. We can hear you	Podemos oirle	(poh-**deh**-mohs oh-**eer**-leh)
17. Put your arms above your head	Ponga sus brazos sobre su cabeza	(**pohn**-gah soos **brah**-sohs **soh**-breh soo kah-**beh**-sah)
18. Take a breath and hold it	Respire y aguante	(reh-**spee**-reh ee ah-goo-**ahn**-teh)
19. Breathe	Respire	(reh-**speer**-eh)

3. IVP

1. The purpose of this test	El propósito de esta prueba	(ehl proh-**poh**-see-toh deh ehs-tah proo-**eh**-bah)
2. Is to check for kidney stones	Es chequear piedras en el riñón	(ehs cheh-keh-**ahr** pee-**eh**-drahs ehn ehl ree-**nyohn**)
3. Have you ever had a kidney stone?	¿Ha tenido alguna vez piedras en el riñón?	(ah teh-**nee**-doh ahl-**goo**-nah vehs pee-**eh**-drahs ehn ehl ree-**nyohn**)
4. Is your pain on the right or left?	¿Es su dolor en el lado derecho o izquierdo?	(ehs soo doh-**lohr** ehn ehl **lah**-doh dehr-**eh**-choh oh ees-kee-**ehr**-doh)
5. Did you see blood in your urine?	¿Vio sangre en la orina?	(vee-oh **sahn**-greh ehn lah oh-**re**-nah)
6. Was there blood in your urine when your doctor tested it?	¿Tuvo sangre en la orina cuando el doctor hizo la prueba?	(too-voh **sahn**-greh ehn lah oh-**ree**-nah koo-**ahn**-doh ehl dohk-**tohr** ee-soh lah proo-**eh**-bah)
7. Are you allergic to contrast?	¿Es usted alérgico a tinta de radiografías?	(ehs oos-**tehd** ah-**lehr**-hee-koh ah **teen**-tah deh rah-dee-oh-grah-**fee**-ahs)
8. What happens?	¿Qué occure?	(keh oh-**kehr**-eh)
9. You need to have an IV	Necesita una línea intravenosa	(neh-seh-**see**-tah oon-ah **leen**-eh-ah een-trah-veh-**noh**-sah)
10. Make a fist	Haga un puño	(ah-gah oon poo-**nyoh**)
11. Now I will inject contrast and then take x-rays	Ahora, le voy a inyectar tinta y tomar radiografías	(ah-**ohr**-ah leh voy ah een-yehk-**tahr** teen-tah ee toh-**mahr** rah-dee-oh-grah-**fee**-ahs)

12.	You can go to the bathroom now	Puede ir al baño ahora	(poo-**eh**-deh eer ahl bah-**nyoh** ah-**ohr**-ah)
13.	Then we will need to take another x-ray	Entonces necesitará otra radiografía	(ehn-**tohn**-sehs neh-seh-see-tahr-**ah** oh-trah rah-dee-oh-grah-**fee**-ah)

4. VCUG

1.	Have you had a urine infection?	¿Ha tenido infección en la orina?	(ah teh-**nee**-doh een-fehk-see-**ohn** ehn lah oh-**ree**-nah)
2.	How many times?	¿Cuántas veces?	(koo-**ahn**-tahs veh-sehs)
3.	We need to put a catheter into the bladder	Necesitamos poner un catéter en la vejiga	(neh-seh-see-**tah**-mohs poh-**neer** oon kah-**teh**-tehr ehn lah veh-**hee**-gah)
4.	The contrast is going in	La tinta está entrando	(lah teen-tah ehs-**tah** ehn-**trahn**-doh)
5.	Turn to the right	Virese a la derecha	(veer-**eh**-seh ah lah dehr-**eh**-chah)
6.	Turn to the left	Virese a la izquierda	(veer-**eh**-seh ah lah ees-kee-**ehr**-dah)
7.	Do you have to urinate?	¿Necesita orinar?	(neh-seh-**see**-tah ohr-ee-**nahr**)
8.	It is important that you tell us when you need to urinate	Es importante que nos diga cuando necesita orinar	(ehs eem-pohr-**tahn**-teh keh nohs **dee**-gah koo-**ahn**-doh neh-seh-**see**-tah oh-ree-**nahr**)
9.	The catheter is out	El catéter está fuera	(ehl kah-**teh**-tehr ehs-**tah** foo-**ehr**-ah)
10.	Urinate into this container	Orine en este recipiente	(ohr-**ee**-neh ehn ehs-teh reh-see-pee-**ehn**-teh)

11. A little bit more	Un poco más	(oon poh-koh **mahs**)
12. That is all	Eso es todo	(**eh**-soh ehs **toh**-doh)

5. MAMMOGRAM (MMG)

1. You are here for a mammogram	Está aquí para una mamografía	(ehs-**tah** ah-**kee** pah-rah oon-ah mah-moh-grah-**fee**-ah)
2. Has anyone in your family had breast cancer?	¿Ha tenido alguien en su familia cáncer del seno?	(ah teh-**nee**-doh ahl-goo-**ee**-ehn ehn soo fah-mee-**lee**-ah **kahn**-sehr dehl **seh**-noh)
3. Grandmother, mother, sister or aunt?	¿Abuela, madre, hermana o tía?	(ah-boo-**eh**-lah, **mah**-dreh, ehr-**mah**-nah, oh **tee**-ah)
4. Why did your doctor send you for this test?	¿Porqué su doctor solicitó esta prueba?	(pohr-**keh** soo dohk-**tohr** soh-lee-see-**toh** ehs-tah proo-**eh**-bah)
5. Routine screening?	¿Para un análisis rutinario?	(pah-rah oon ah-**nah**-lee-sees roo-tee-nahr-**ee**-oh)
6. Did you feel a lump in the breast?	¿Sintió un bulto en el seno?	(seen-tee-**oh** oon **bool**-toh ehn ehl **seh**-noh)
7. Did your doctor feel a lump?	¿Sintió su doctor un bulto?	(seen-tee-**oh** soo dohk-**tohr** oon **bool**-toh)
8. Do you have pain?	¿Tiene dolor?	(tee-**ehn**-eh doh-**lohr**)
9. Which side? Right or left?	¿De qué lado? ¿Derecho o izquierdo?	(deh **keh** lah-doh deh-reh-choh oh ees-kee-ehr-doh)
10. Have you ever had a MMg?	¿Ha tenido algúna vez una mamografía?	(ah teh-**nee**-doh ahl-**goo**-nah vehs oon-ah mah-moh-grah-**fee**-ah)

11. Here?	¿Aquí?	(ah-**kee**)
12. At what hospital?	¿En qué hospital?	(ehn **keh** ohs-pee-**tahl**)
13. When?	¿Cuándo?	(koo-**ahn**-doh)
14. Sit here	Siéntese aquí	(see-**ehn**-teh-seh ah-**kee**)
15. Do not move	No se mueva	(noh seh moo-**eh**-vah)
16. You need to have an ultrasound	Necesita un ultrasonido	(neh-seh-**see**-tah oon ool-trah-sohn-**ee**-doh)
17. You probably have a cyst	Probablemente tiene un quiste	(proh-bah-bleh-**mehn**-teh tee-**eh**-neh oon **kees**-teh)
18. However, it could be something else	Sin embargo, puede ser otra cosa	(seen ehm-**bahr**-goh poo-**eh**-deh sehr oh-trah **koh**-sah)
19. Lie down here	Acuéstese aquí	(ah-koo-**ehs**-teh-sah ah-**kee**)
20. It is a cyst	Es un quiste	(ehs oon **kees**-teh)
21. Return here in 1 year for a follow up MMg	Regrese aquí en un año para su próxima mammografía	(reh-**greh**-seh ah-**kee** ehn oon ah-**nyoh** pah-rah soo **prohx**-ee-mah mah-moh-grah-**fee**-ah)
22. You need to have a biopsy	Necesita una biopsia	(neh-seh-**see**-tah oon-ah bee-ohp-**see**-ah)
23. You have a group of calcifications in the left breast	Tiene un grupo de calcificaciones en el seno izquierdo	(tee-**ehn**-eh oon **groo**-poh deh kahl-see-fee-kah-see-**ohn**-ehs ehn ehl **seh**-noh ees-kee-**ehr**-doh)
24. Which are probably benign	Probablemente son benigno	(proh-bah-bleh-**mehn**-teh sohn beh-**neeg**-noh)
25. However, these calcifications could be an early sign of malignancy	Sin embargo estas calcificaciones pueden ser una señal de malignidad	(seen ehm-**bahr**-goh ehs-tahs kahl-see-fee-kah-see-**ohn**-ehs poo-**eh**-dehn sehr oon-ah seh-**nyahl** deh mah-leeg-nee-**dahd**)

6. MAGNETIC RESONANCE IMAGING (MRI)

1. MRI images are very detailed	Las imagenes de resonancia magnética son muy detalladas	(lahs ee-mah-**heh**-nehs deh re-soh-nahn-**see**-ah mahg-**neh**-tee-kah sohn moo-ee deh-tah-**yah**-dahs)
2. MRI is especially helpful for diseases and injuries	MRI es especialmente útil para enfermedades y golpes	(MRI ehs ehs-peh-see-ahl-**mehn**-teh **oo**-teel pah-rah ehn-fehr-mee-**dah**-dehs ee **gohl**-pehs)
3. Of the brain, spine, liver, knees and hips	Del cerebro, espinazo, hígado, rodillas y caderas	(dehl sehr-**eh**-broh, ehs-pee-**nah**-soh, **ee**-gah-doh, roh-**dee**-yahs ee kah-**dehr**-ahs)
4. You will lie down on a table	Usted se acostará en una mesa	(oos-**tehd** seh ah-kohs-tahr-**ah** ehn oon-ah **meh**-sah)
5. A giant magnet shaped like a doughnut will surround you	Un imán grande como una rosca le rodeará	(oon ee-**mahn grahn**-deh koh-moh oon-ah **rohs**-kah leh roh-deh-ahr-**ah**)
6. If you have claustrophobia	Si tiene claustrofobia	(see tee-**eh**-neh klah-oos-troh-foh-**bee**-ah)
7. We can give you medicine to help you relax	Podemos darle alguna medicina para calmarle	(poh-**deh**-mohs **dahr**-leh ahl-**goo**-nah meh-dee-**see**-nah pah-rah kahl-**mahr**-leh)
8. Did you come here with anyone?	¿Vino usted con alguien?	(vee-noh oos-**tehd** kohn ahl-goo-**ee**-ehn)
9. Can this person drive you home?	¿Puede esta persona manejar el coche?	(poo-**eh**-deh ehs-tah pehr-**sohn**-ah mahn-eh-**hahr** ehl **koh**-cheh)
10. Do you want the medicine?	¿Quiere la medicina?	(kee-**ehr**-eh lah meh-dee-**see**-nah)

11. You cannot drive for the rest of today	No puede manejar el coche por el resto de día	(noh poo-**eh**-deh mahn-eh-**hahr** ehl **koh**-cheh pohr ehl rehs-toh deh **dee**-ah)
12. Do you have a pacemaker?	¿Tiene usted un marcapasos?	(tee-**eh**-neh oo-**stehd** oon mahr-kah-**pah**-sohs)
13. Have you ever had an aneurysm in your brain?	¿Ha tenido algún aneurisma en su cerebro?	(ah teh-**nee**-doh ahl-**goon** ahn-eh-oor-**ees**-mah ehn soo sehr-**eh**-broh)
14. Did you have surgery?	¿Tuvo cirugía?	(too-voh see-roo-**hee**-ah)
15. Is it possible that you have a piece of metal in your eye?	¿Es posible que usted tenga un pedazo de metal en el ojo?	(ehs poh-**see**-bleh keh oos-**tehd** tehn-gah oon peh-**dah**-soh deh meh-**tahl** ehn ehl **oh**-hoh)
16. Do you have a neurostimulator?	¿Tiene usted una máquina para estimular los nervios?	(tee-**eh**-neh oos-**tehd** oon-ah **mah**-kee-nah pah-rah ehs-tee-moo-**lahr** lohs nehr-**vee**-ohs)
17. Do you have a cochlear implant?	¿Tiene un implante coclear?	(tee-**ehn**-eh oon eem-**plahn**-teh koh-kleh-**ahr**)
18. Do you have any artificial valves in your heart?	¿Tiene alguna valvula artificial en su corazón?	(tee-**eh**-neh ahl-**goo**-nah **vahl**-voo-lah ehr-tee-fee-see-**ahl** ehn soo kohr-ah-**sohn**)
19. Are you pregnant?	¿Está embarazada?	(ehs-**tah** ehm-vahr-ah-**sah**-dah)
20. Are you sure?	¿Está segura?	(ehs-**tah** seh-**goo**-rah)
21. MRI does not use x-rays	MRI no usa rayos x	(MRI noh **oos**-ah **rah**-yohs eh-kees)

7. NUCLEAR MEDICINE

V/Q SCAN

1. The purpose of this test	El propósito de esta prueba	(ehl proh-**poh**-see-toh deh ehs-tah proo-**eh**-bah)

2. Is to check for a blood clot in your lungs	Es chequear por un coágulo de sangre en los pulmones	(ehs cheh-keh-**ahr** pohr oon koh-**ah**-goo-loh deh **sahn**-greh ehn lohs pool-**mohn**-ehs)
3. Sit here	Siéntese aquí	(see-**ehn**-teh-seh ah-**kee**)
4. You need to wear this mask	Necesita usar esta máscara	(neh-seh-**see**-tah oo-**sahr** ehs-tah **mahs**-kahr-ah)
5. Breathe	Respire	(reh-**spee**-reh)
6. Relax	Relájese	(reh-**lah**-heh-seh)
7. You need to have an IV	Necesita una línea intravenosa	(neh-seh-**see**-tah oon-ah **leen**-eh-ah een-trah-vehn-**oh**-sah)
8. Lie down	Acuéstese	(ah-koo-**ehs**-teh-seh)
9. Make a fist	Haga un puño	(**ah**-gah oon poo-**nyoh**)
10. You will feel a little stick	Sentirá un pinchazo	(sehn-eer-**ah** oon peen-**chah**-soh)
11. This chemical goes to the lungs and helps to show clots	Este químico va a los pulmones y ayuda a detectar coágulos	(ehs-teh **kee**-mee-koh vah ah lohs pool-**mohn**-ehs ee eye-**oo**-dah ah deh-tehk-**tahr** koh-**ah**-goo-lohs)
12. This camera will take the picture	Esta cámara tomará la radiografía	(ehs-tah **kah**-mahr-ah toh-mahr-**ah** lah rah-dee-**oh**-grah-**fee**-ah)
13. Try not to move	No se mueva	(noh seh moo-**eh**-vah)

HIDA SCAN

1. The purpose of this test	El propósito de esta prueba	(ehl proh-**poh**-see-toh deh ehs-tah proo-**eh**-bah)
2. Is to check for inflammation of the gallbladder	Es chequear inflamación en la vesícula biliar	(ehs cheh-keh-**ahr** een-flah-mah-see-**ohn** ehn lah veh-**see**-koo-lah vee-lee-**ahr**)

3. Caused by obstruction by a stone	Causada por una obstrucción de piedra	(kah-oo-**sah**-dah pohr oon-ah ohbs-trook-see-**ohn** deh pee-**ehr**-dah)
4. When was your last meal?	¿Cuándo fue su última comida?	(koo-**ahn**-doh foo-**eh** soo **ool**-tee-mah koh-**mee**-dah)
5. Usually this test takes 1 to 4 hours	Usualmente la prueba tarda de una o cuatro horas	(oos-oo-ahl-**mehn**-teh lah proo-**eh**-bah **tahr**-dah de oon-ah oh koo-**ah**-troh **ohr**-ahs)
6. Normally this chemical goes to the gallbladder and bowel	Normalmente este químico va a la vesícula biliar y el intestino	(nohr-mahl-**mehn**-teh esh-teh **kee**-mee-koh vah ah lah veh-**see**-koo-lah bee-lee-**ahr** ee ehl een-tehs-**tee**-noh)
7. If the gallbladder is blocked	Si la vesícula biliar está bloqueada	(see lah veh-**see**-koo-lah bee-lee-**ahr** ehs-**tah** bloh-keh-**ah**-dah)
8. The chemical will only go to the intestine	El químico solamente va al intestino	(ehl **kee**-mee-koh soh-lah-**mehn**-teh vah ahl een-tehs-**tee**-noh)
9. Did you have a U/S of the gallbladder?	¿Tuvo un ultrasonido de la vesícula biliar?	(too-voh oon ool-trah-sohn-**ee**-doh deh lah veh-**see**-koo-lah bee-lee-**ahr**)

BONE SCAN

1. The purpose of this test	El propósito de esta prueba	(ehl proh-**poh**-see-toh deh ehs-tah proo-**eh**-bah)
2. Is to check for a fracture, infection or tumor	Es chequear por una fractura, infección o tumor	(ehs cheh-keh-**ahr** pohr oon-ah frahk-**too**-rah een-fehk-see-**ohn** oh too-**mohr**)
3. A small amount of a radioactive chemical	Una pequeña cantidad de químico radióactivo	(oon-ah peh-keh-**nyah** kahn-tee-**dahd** deh **kee**-mee-koh rah-dee-**oh**-ahk-tee-voh)
4. will be injected into your arm	será inyectado en su brazo	(seh-**rah** een-yehk-**tah**-doh ehn soo **brah**-soh)

5. The amount of radiation is similar to that of several x-rays	La cantidad de radiación es la misma que la de algunas radiografías	(lah kahn-tee-**dahd** deh rah-dee-ah-see-**ohn** ehs lah **mees**-mah keh lah deh ahl-**goo**-nahs rah-dee-oh-grah-**fee**-ahs)
6. In 2 to 4 hours the pictures will be taken	En dos o cuatro horas se tomarán las radiografías	(ehn dohs oh koo-ah-troh **ohr**-ahs seh toh-mah-**rahn** lahs rah-dee-oh-grah-**fee**-ahs)
7. You should drink a lot of water	Debe tomar mucha agua	(deh-beh toh-**mahr** moo-chah ah-**goo**-ah)
8. This helps to more quickly remove the chemical from your body	Esto ayuda a remover el químico de su cuerpo más rápido	(ehs-toh eye-**oo**-dah ah reh-moh-**vehr** ehl **kee**-mee-koh de soo koo-**ehr**-poh **mahs rah**-pee-doh)

8. ULTRASOUND GENERAL INFORMATION

1. What is your name?	¿Cómo se llama?	(**koh**-moh seh **yah**-mah)
2. Hi, my name is	Hola, mi nombre es	(**oh**-lah mee **nohm**-breh ehs)
3. I will be doing your ultrasound	Yo le haré su ultrasonido	(yoh leh ahr-**eh** soo ool-trah-sohn-**ee**-doh)
4. Do you speak English?	¿Habla inglés?	(ah-blah een-**glehs**)
5. I only speak a little Spanish	Sólo hablo un poquito de español	(**soh**-loh **ah**-bloh oon poh-**kee**-toh deh ehs-pah-**nyohl**)
6. Please speak very slowly	Por favor hable despacio	(pohr fah-**vohr** ah-bleh dehs-**pah**-see-oh)
7. Say that again please	Otra vez por favor	(**oh**-trah vehs pohr fah-**vohr**)
8. Have you ever had an U/S in the past?	¿Ha tenido un ultrasonido en el pasado?	(ah teh-**nee**-doh oon ool-trah-sohn-**ee**-doh ehn ehl pah-**sah**-doh)

9.	What part of the body?	¿En qué parte del cuerpo?	(ehn **keh** pahr-teh dehl koo-**ehr**-poh)
10.	In this hospital?	¿En este hospital?	(ehn ehs-teh ohs-pee-**tahl**)
11.	In what hospital?	¿En qué hospital?	(ehn **keh** ohs-pee-**tahl**)
12.	When?	¿Cuándo?	(koo-**ahn**-doh)
13.	Was it normal?	¿Fue normal?	(foo-eh nohr-**mahl**)
14.	What were the results?	¿Cuáles fueron los resultados?	(koo-**ahl**-ehs foo-**ehr**-ohn lohs reh-sool-**tah**-dohs)
15.	We will not use any needles	No usaremos agujas	(noh oo-sahr-**eh**-mohs ah-**goo**-hahs)
16.	The results of this test	Los resultados de esta prueba	(lohs reh-sool-**tah**-dohs deh ehs-tah proo-**eh**-bah)
17.	Will help determine which treatment is best for you	Ayudarán a determinar el tratamiento mejor para usted	(eye-oo-dahr-**ahn** ah deh-tehr-meen-**ahr** ehl trah-tah-mee-**ehn**-toh meh-**hohr** pah-rah oos-**tehd**)
18.	Please come with me	Por favor venga conmigo	(pohr fah-**vohr** vehn-gah kohn-**mee**-goh)
19.	Please lie down on this table/bed	Por favor acuéstese en está cama	(pohr fah-**vohr** ah-koo-**ehs**-teh-seh ehn ehs-tah **kah**-mah)
20.	Are you o.k.?	¿Está bien?	(ehs-**tah** bee-**ehn**)
21.	Are you short of breath?	¿Tiene dificultad al respirar?	(tee-**eh**-neh dee-fee-kool-**tahd** ahl rehs-peer-**ahr**)
22.	Would another pillow help?	¿Quiere otra almohada?	(kee-ehr-eh oh-trah ahl-moh-**ah**-dah)
23.	Here is a towel to help protect your clothes from the gel	Aquí tiene una toalla para proteger su ropa de la gelatina	(ah-**kee** tee-**ehn**-eh oon-ah toh-**ah**-yah pah-rah proh-teh-**hehr** soo roh-pah deh lah heh-lah-**teen**-ah)

24. Where does it hurt the most?	¿Dónde le duele más?	(**dohn**-deh leh doo-**eh**-leh **mahs**)
25. Please show me with one finger	Por favor enséñeme con un dedo	(pohr fah-**vohr** ehn-**seh**-nyeh-meh kohn oon **deh**-doh)
26. Hold your breath	Aguante la respiración	(ah-goo-**ahn**-teh lah rehs-peer-ah-see-**ohn**)
27. Stop breathing	No respire	(noh rehs-**peer**-eh)
28. Breathe	Respire	(rehs-**peer**-eh)
29. Please, try not to move	Por favor no se mueva	(pohr fah-**vohr** noh seh moo-**eh**-vah)
30. So far everything looks normal	Por ahora todo se ve normal	(pohr ah-**ohr**-ah toh-doh seh veh nohr-**mahl**)
31. We are almost finished	Casi terminamos	(kah-see tehr-mee-**nah**-mohs)
32. That is all	Esto es todo	(ehs-toh ehs **toh**-doh)
33. Here is a towel to remove the gel	Aquí tiene una toalla para remover la gelatina	(ah-kee tee-**ehn**-eh oon-ah toh-**ah**-yah pah-rah reh-moh-**vehr** lah heh-lah-**tee**-nah)
34. Wait here	Espere aquí	(ehs-**peer**-eh ah-**kee**)
35. Wait in the room by the receptionist	Espere en la sala cerca de la recepcionista	(ehs-**peer**-eh ehn lah **sah**-lah **sehr**-kah deh lah reh-sehp-see-ohn-**ees**-tah)
36. I am going to call your doctor	Voy a llamar a su doctor	(voh-ee ah yah-**mahr** ah soo dohk-**tohr**)
37. Your doctor will discuss the results with you	El doctor discutirá los resultados con usted	(ehl dohk-**tohr** dees-koo-teer-**ah** lohs reh-sool-**tah**-dohs kohn oos-**tehd**)
38. I will return in a few minutes	Regreso en unos minutos	(reh-**greh**-soh ehn oon-ohs mee-**noo**-tohs)

39. Do you have an appointment with your doctor today?	¿Tiene una cita con su doctor hoy?	(tee-**eh**-neh oon-ah **see**-tah kohn soo dohk-**tohr** oy)
40. You need to talk to the receptionist before you go	Necesita hablar con la recepcionista antes de irse	(neh-seh-**see**-tah ah-**blahr** kohn lah reh-sehp-see-ohn-**ees**-tah ahn-tehs deh **eer**-seh)
41. You can go	Puede irse	(poo-**eh**-deh **eer**-seh)
42. Take care	Cuidese	(koo-ee-**deh**-seh)

9. OBSTETRIC ULTRASOUND

1. When was your last menstrual period?	¿Cuándo fue su última regla?	(koo-**ahn**-doh foo-eh soo **ool**-tee-mah **reh**-glah)
2. Was that the first day?	¿Fue ese el primer día?	(foo-eh ehs-eh ehl pree-mehr **dee**-ah)
3. Are you sure?	¿Está segura?	(ehs-**tah** seh-**goo**-rah)
4. When is your due date?	¿Cuál es la fecha del nacimiento?	(koo-**ahl** ehs lah **feh**-chah deh nah-see-mee-**ehn**-toh)
5. Have you had any other ultrasounds during this pregnancy?	¿Ha tenido otro ultrosonido durante este embarazo?	(ah teh-**nee**-doh oh-troh ool-troh-sohn-**ee**-doh doo-**rahn**-teh ehs-teh ehm-bahr-**ar**-soh)
6. When?	¿Cuándo?	(koo-**ahn**-doh)
7. Where?	¿Dónde?	(**dohn**-deh)
8. Do you want to know if its a boy or girl?	¿Quiere saber si es un niño o niña?	(kee-**ehr**-eh sah-**behr** see ehs oon nee-**nyoh** oh nee-**nyah**)
9. You may lie on your side if you feel uncomfortable	Puede acostarse sobre su lado si se siente incómoda	(poo-**eh**-deh ah-koh-**stahr**-seh soh-breh soo **lah**-doh see seh see-**ehn**-teh een-**koh**-moh-dah)

10.	I'm sorry, I need to push a little bit	Lo siento pero necesito empujar un poco	(loh see-**ehn**-toh pehr-oh neh-seh-**see**-toh ehm-poo-**hahr** oon **poh**-koh)
11.	Do you have any other children?	¿Tiene otros hijos?	(tee-**ehn**-eh oh-trohs **ee**-hohs)
12.	Did you have any problems with your pregnancies?	¿Tuvo algúnos problemás con sus otros embarazos?	(too-voh ahl-**goo**-nohs proh-bleh-**mahs** kohn soos **oh**-trohs ehm-bahr-**ah**-sohs)
13.	It is a boy (probably)	Es un niño, probablemente	(ehs oon **nee**-nyoh proh-bah-blah-**mehn**-teh)
14.	It is a girl (probably)	Es una niña, probablemente	(ehs oon-ah **nee**-nyah proh-bah-bleh-**mehn**-teh)
15.	We are almost finished	Casi terminamos	(kah-see tehr-mee-**nah**-mohs)

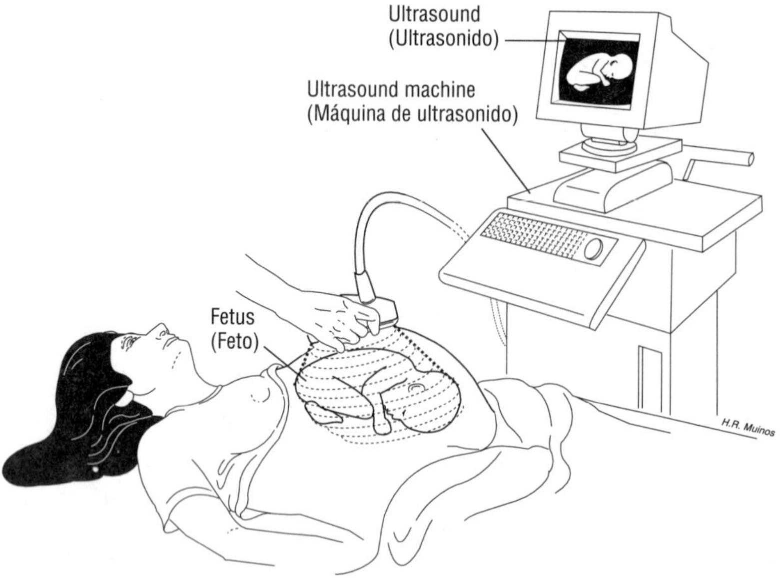

Figure 1. Ultrasound with fetus.

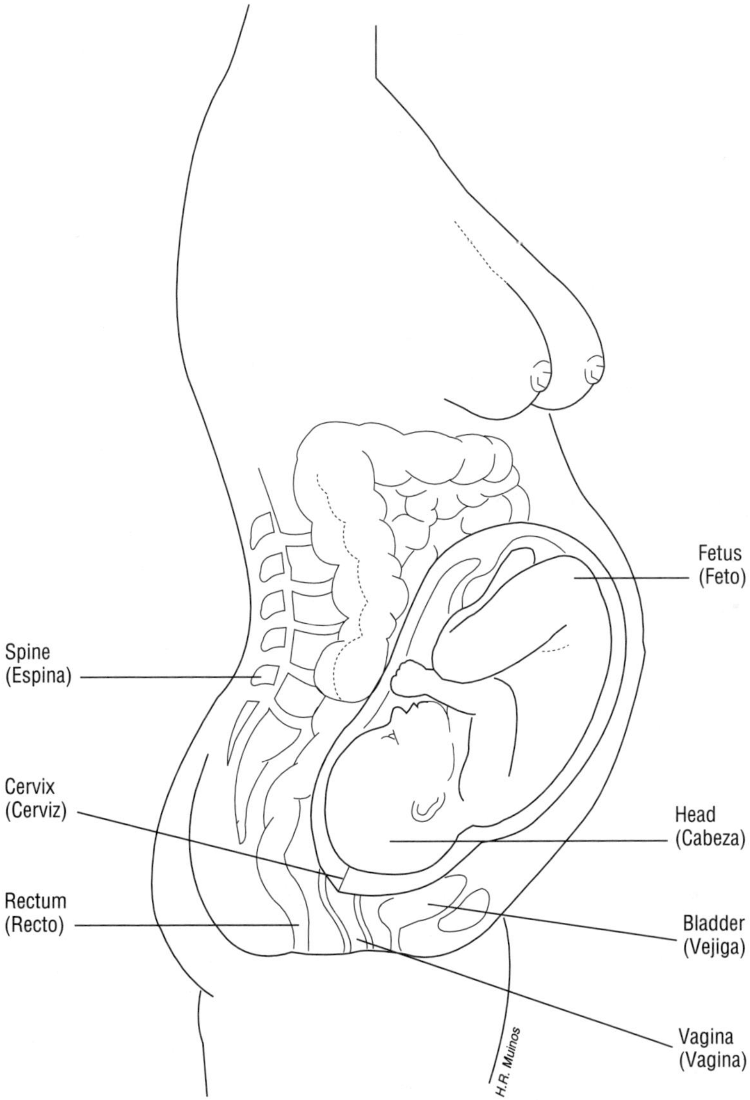

Figure 2. Female with 9-month fetus.

16.	You should return here for another ultrasound in 4 weeks	Debe regresar aquí para otro ultrasonido en cuatro semanas	(deh-beh reh-greh-**sahr** ah-**kee** pah-rah oh-troh ool-trah-sohn-**ee**-doh ehn koo-**ah**-troh seh-**mahn**-ahs)
17.	At 9:00 in the morning	A las nueve de la mañana	(ah lahs noo-**eh**-veh deh lah mah-**nyah**-nah)
18.	At 2:00 in the afternoon	A las dos de la tarde	(ah lahs dohs deh lah **tahr**-deh)

10. ENDOVAGINAL ULTRASOUND

1.	The best type of U/S for your condition is endovaginal	El mejor tipo de ultrasonido para su condición es el endovaginal	(ehl meh-**hohr** tee-poh deh ool-trah-sohn-**ee**-doh pah-rah soo kohn-dee-see-**ohn** ehs ehl ehn-doh-vah-hee-**nahl**)
2.	When the U/S transducer is in the vagina	Cuando el transductor del ultrasonido está en la vagina	(koo-**ahn**-doh ehl trahns-dook-**tohr** dehl ool-trah-sohn-**ee**-doh ehs-**tah** ehn lah vah-**hee**-nah)
3.	It is closer to the uterus and ovaries	Está más cerca del útero y de los ovarios	(ehs-**tah mahs** sehr-kah dehl **oo**-tehr-oh ee ah lohs oh-vehr-**ee**-ohs)
4.	Generally it can detect the presence of a baby or fetus	Generalmente puede detectar la presencia de un bebé o feto	(hehn-ehr-ahl-**mehn**-teh poo-**eh**-deh deh-tehk-**tahr** lah preh-sehn-**see**-ah deh oon beh-**beh** oh feh-toh)
5.	One week earlier than regular U/S of the abdomen	Una semana antes del ultrasonido a través del adbomen	(oon-ah seh-**mahn**-ah ahn-tehs dehl ool-trah-sohn-**ee**-doh ah trah-**vehs** dehl ahb-**doh**-mehn)

6. The U/S transducer is smaller than the speculum used by the gynecologist	El transductor es más pequeño que el espéculo usado por el ginecólogo	(ehl trahns-dook-**tohr** ehs mahs peh-**keh**-nyoh keh ehl ehs-**peh**-koo-loh oo-**sah**-doh pah-rah ehl heen-eh-**koh**-loh-goh)
7. This type of U/S is done with the bladder empty	Este tipo de ultrasonido se hace con la vejiga vacía	(ehs-teh **tee**-poh deh ool-tra-sohn-**ee**-doh seh ah-seh kohn lah vee-**hee**-gah vah-**see**-ah)

11. ABDOMINAL ULTRASOUND

1. Where does it hurt more?	¿Dónde le duele más?	(**dohn**-deh le doo-eh-leh **mahs**)
2. Here or here (e.g. while you point to spot)	¿Aquí o aquí?	(ah-**kee** oh ah-**kee**)
3. Since when have you had this pain?	¿Desde cuándo tiene este dolor?	(dehs-deh koo-**ahn**-doh tee-**ehn**-eh ehs-teh doh-**lohr**)
4. Have you ever had this type of pain before?	¿Ha tenido este tipo de dolor anteriormente?	(ah teh-**nee**-doh ehs-teh **tee**-poh deh doh-**lohr** ahn-tehr-ee-ohr-**mehn**-teh)
5. Did you have a fever?	¿Tiene fiebre?	(tee-**ehn**-eh fee-**eh**-breh)

12. LOWER EXTREMITY VENOUS ULTRASOUND

1. You are here for an U/S of the veins in your leg	Usted está aquí para un ultrasonido de las venas en su pierna	(oos-**tehd** ehs-**tah** ah-**kee** pah-rah oon ool-trah-sohn-**ee**-doh deh lahs **vee**-nahs ehn soo pee-**ehr**-nah)

2. The purpose of this test	El propósito de esta prueba	(ehl proh-**poh**-see-toh deh **ehs**-tah proo-**eh**-bah)
3. Is to check for a blood clot in your legs	Es para chequear por coágulos de sangre en sus piernas	(ehs pah-ah cheh-keh-**ahr** pohr koh-**ah**-goo-lohs deh **sahn**-greh ehn soos pee-**ehr**-nahs)
4. Clots from the veins in the leg	Los coágulos en las venas de la pierna	(lohs koh-**ah**-goo-lohs ehn lahs **veh**-nahs deh la pee-**ehr**-nah)
5. Sometimes become loose and go to the lung	A veces se separan y van al pulmón	(ah **veh**-sehs seh seh-pahr-**ahn** ee vahn ahl pool-**mohn**)
6. This can cause shortness of breath, chest pain or coughing	Esto puede causar dificultad al respirar, dolor en el pecho y tos	(ehs-toh poo-**eh**-deh kah-oo-**sahr** dee-fee-kool-**tahd** ahl rehs-peer-**ahr** doh-**lohr** ehn ehl **peh**-choh ee tohs)
7. I need to press down with the transducer to check the veins	Necesito empujar hacia abajo con el transductor para chequear las venas	(neh-seh-**see**-toh ehm-poo-**hahr** ah-see-ah ah-**bah**-hoh kohn ehl trahs-dook-**tohr** pah-rah cheh-keh-**ahr** lahs **veh**-nahs)
8. You have a blood clot in your leg	Tiene un coágulo de sangre en su pierna	(tee-**ehn**-eh oon koh-**ah**-goo-loh deh **sahn**-greh ehn soo pee-**ehr**-nah)
9. Usually, the treatment is medicines to help dissolve the clot	Usualmente, el tratamiento es usar medicinas para ayudar a disolver el coágulo	(oos-oo-ahl-**mehn**-teh, ehl trah-tah-mee-**ehn**-toh ehs oo-**sahr** meh-dee-**see**-nahs pah-rah eye-oo-**dahr** ah dee-sohl-**vehr** ehl koh-**ah**-goo-loh)

13. LOWER EXTREMITY ARTERIAL ULTRASOUND

1. Do you have pain in your leg?	¿Tiene dolor en la pierna?	(tee-**ehn**-eh doh-**lohr** ehn lah pee-**ehr**-nah)

2. Right, left, or both	¿Derecha, izquierda, o ambas?	(dehr-**eh**-chah, ees-kee-**ehr**-dah oh **ahm**-bahs)
3. Which side is worse?	¿Qué lado es peor?	(**keh** lah-doh ehs peh-**ohr**)
4. Do you have pain when you walk?	¿Le duele cuándo camina?	(leh doo-**eh**-leh koo-**ahn**-doh kah-**mee**-nah)
5. Is it always the same distance?	¿Es siempre la misma distancia?	(ehs see-**ehm**-preh la **mees**-mah dees-tahn-**see**-ah)
6. One or two blocks?	¿Una o dos cuadras?	(oon-ah oh dohs koo-**ah**-drahs)
7. The purpose of this test	El propósito de esta prueba	(ehl proh-**poh**-see-toh deh ehs-tah proo-**eh**-bah)
8. Is to check for narrowing or blockage in the arteries of the leg	Es para chequear la estrechez o bloqueo de las arterias de la pierna	(esh pah-rah cheh-keh-**ahr** lah ehs-treh-**chehs** oh bloh-**keh**-oh deh lahs ahr-tehr-**ee** lahs deh lah pee-**ehr**-nah)
9. I need to take the blood pressure in your leg	Necesito tomar la presión en su pierna	(neh-seh-see-toh toh-mahr lah preh-see-**ohn** ehn soo pee-ehr-nah)

14. PLAIN FILM X-RAYS

1. Lie down	Acuéstese	(ah-koo-**ehs**-teh-seh)
2. Sit up	Siéntese	(see-**ehn**-teh-seh)
3. Stand up	Párese	(**pahr**-eh-seh)
4. Take a deep breath and hold it	Respire profundamente y aguántelo	(reh-**spee**-reh proh-foon-dah-**mehn**-teh ee ah-goo-**ahn**-teh-loh)

5. Breathe	Respire	(rehs-**pee**-reh)
6. Put your hands above your head	Ponga sus manos sobre la cabeza	(pohn-gah soos **mah**-nohs soh-breh lah kah-**beh**-sah)
7. Do not move	No se mueva	(noh seh moo-**eh**-vah)

Section Seven

IMAGING GUIDED PROCEDURES

CHAPTER OUTLINE

1. ARTERIOGRAPHY GENERAL INFORMATION

1. You are here for an arteriogram	Usted esta aquí para un arteriograma	(oos-tehd ehs-tah ah-**kee** pah-rah oon ahr-tehr-ee-o-**grah**-mah)
2. Your doctor(s) asked us to do this test to check for narrowing in the arteries	Su doctor solicitó esta prueba para chequear la estrechez de las arterias	(soo dohk-**tohr** soh-lee-see-**toh** ehs-tah proo-**eh**-bah pah-rah cheh-keh-**ahr** lah ehs-treh-**chehs** deh lahs ahr-tehr-**ee**-ahs)
3. For this procedure we will put a catheter into the artery near the hip	Para este procedimiento pondremos un catéter dentro de la arteria de la cadera	(pah-rah ehs-teh proh-see-dee-mee-**ehn**-toh pohn-**dreh**-mohs oon kah-**teh**-tehr dehn-troh deh lah ahr-tehr-**ee**-ah deh lah kah-**dehr**-ah)
4. We will then position the catheter in the aorta	Entonces colocaremos el catéter en la aorta	(ehn-**tohn**-sehs koh-loh-kahr-**eh**-mohs ehl kah-**teh**-tehr ehn lah ah-**ohr**-tah)
5. And inject contrast (x-ray dye)	E inyectaremos tinta	(eh een-yehk-tahr-**eh**-mohs **teen**-tah)

6. We will need to take several sets of radiographs	Necesitaremos tomarle varios grupos de radiografías	(neh-seh-see-tahr-**eh**-mohs toh-**mahr**-leh vahr-**ee**-ohs groo-pohs deh rah-dee-oh-grah-**fee**-ahs)
7. Then we will remove the catheter	Entonces, sacaremos el catéter	(ehn-**tohn**-sehs, sah-kahr-**eh**-mohs ehl kah-**teh**-tehr)
8. We will hold pressure on this spot for 10 to 15 minutes	Pondremos presión en este lugar por diez o quince minutos	(pohn-**dreh**-mohs preh-see-**ohn** ehn ehs-teh loo-**gahr** pohr dee-ehs oh **keen**-seh mee-**noo**-tohs)
9. You will need to stay in bed and keep your leg straight for 6 hours	Necesitará quedarse en la cama durante seis horas con las piernas estiradas	(neh-seh-see-tahr-**ah** keh-**dahr**-seh ehn lah **kah**-mah doo-**rahn**-teh seh-ees **ohr**-ahs kohn lahs pee-**ehr**-nahs ehs-teer-**ah**-dahs)
10. This procedure is very common	Este procedimiento es muy común	(ehs-teh proh-seh-dee-mee-**ehn**-toh ehs moo-ee koh-**moon**)
11. We do this procedure 3 times a day	Nosotros hacemos este procedimiento tres veces al día	(noh-**soh**-trohs ah-**seh**-mohs ehs-teh proh-seh-dee-mee-**ehn**-toh trehs veh-sehs ahl **dee**-ah)
12. I will give you local anesthesia	Yo le daré anestesia local	(yoh leh dahr-**eh** ahn-ehs-teh-**see**-ah loh-**kahl**)
13. If you have any pain	Si tiene algún dolor	(see tee-**ehn**-eh ahl-**goon** doh-**lohr**)
14. Tell us and we will give you more pain medicines	Déjenos saber y le daremos más medicina para el dolor	(**deh**-heh-nohs sah-**behr** ee leh dahr-**eh**-mohs **mahs** meh-dee-**see**-nah pah-rah ehl doh-**lohr**)
15. We can also give you medicine in your IV to help prevent discomfort	También podemos darle algunas medicina en el suero para evitar molestia	(tahm-bee-**ehn** poh-**deh**-mohs dahr-leh ahl-**goo**-nahs meh-dee-**see**-nah ehn ehl soo-**ehr**-oh pah-rah eh-vee-**tahr** moh-lehs-**tee**-ah)

16.	However, you need to be awake during the procedure	Sin embargo, necesitará mantenerse despierto durante el procedimiento	(seen ehm-**bahr**-goh, neh-seh-see-tahr-**ah** mahn-teh-**nehr**-seh dehs-pee-**ehr**-toh doo-**rahn**-teh ehl proh-seh-dee-mee-**ehn**-toh)
17.	Because you will need to hold your breath at certain times	Porque usted necesitará aguantar su respiración en ciertos momentos	(pohr keh oos-**tehd** neh-seh-see-tahr-**ah** ah-goo-ahn-**tahr** soo rehs-pee-rah-see-**ohn** ehn see **ehr** tohs moh-**mehn**-tohs)
18.	And we need to be able to talk to you	Y necesitaremos hablar con usted	(ee neh-seh-see-tahr-**eh**-mohs ah-**blahr** kohn oos-**tehd**)

2. ARTERIOGRAPHY INFORMED CONSENT

1.	The most common problem is bleeding where the needle goes into the artery	El problema más común es hemorragia, donde la aguja entra en la arteria	(ehl proh-**bleh**-mah **mahs** koh-**moon** ehs ehm-ohr-ah-**hee**-ah, dohn-deh lah ah-**goo**-hah ehn-trah ehn lah ahr-tehr-**ee**-ah)
2.	If this occurs we will stop it by putting pressure over the artery	Si esto ocurre la detendremos poniendo presión sobre la arteria	(see ehs-toh oh-**koo**-reh lah deh-tehn-**dreh**-mohs pohn-ee-**ehn**-doh preh-see-**ohn** soh-breh lah ahr-tehr-**ee**-ah)
3.	The amount of bleeding usually is not significant	Usualmente la cantidad de sangre no es significartivo	(oos-oo-ahl-**mehn**-teh lah kahn-tee-**dahd** deh **sahn**-greh noh ehs seeg-nee-fee-kahr-**tee**-voh)
4.	Less than 1 out of 100 persons will need a blood transfusion	Menos de una en cada cien personas necesitará transfusión de sangre	(meh-nohs deh oon-ah ehn **kah**-dah see-ehn pehr-**soh**-nahs neh-seh-see-tahr-**ah** trahns-foo-see-**ohn** deh **sahn**-gre)

5. Also, 1 out of 100 persons (more or less) has the risk of injury to the arteries	También, una en cada cien personas tiene el riesgo de lastimarse las arterias	(tahm-bee-**ehn**, oon-ah ehn kah-dah see-ehn pehr-**soh**-nahs tee-**ehn**-eh ehl ree-**ehs**-goh deh lahs-tee-**mahr**-seh lahs ahr-tehr-**ee**-ahs)
6. Especially the artery by the hip	Especialmente la arteria cerca de la cadera	(ehs-peh-see-ahl-**mehn**-teh lah ahr-tehr-**ee**-ah sehr-kah deh lah kah-**dehr**-ah)
7. The artery sometimes develops an abnormal bulge	A veces la arteria desarrolla un bulto anormal	(ah veh-sehs lah ahr-tehr-**ee**-ah deh-sahr-**oh**-yah oon **bool**-toh ah-nohr-**mahl**)
8. This is called a pseudoaneurysm	Esto se llama un pseudoaneurisma	(ehs-toh seh **yah**-mah oon seh-oo-doh-ah-neh-oo-**rees**-mah)
9. It can be seen on U/S	Se puede ver en el ultrasonido	(seh poo-**eh**-deh vehr ehn ehl ool-trah-sohn-**ee**-doh)
10. Usually it is treated by compression with the ultrasound transducer	Usualmente el tratamiento es compresión con el transductor del ultrasonido	(oo-soo-ahl-**mehn**-teh ehl trah-tah-mee-**ehn**-toh ehs kohm-preh-see-**ohn** kohn ehl trahns-dook-**tohr** dehl ool-trah-soh-**nee**-doh)
11. Sometimes the surgeon will need to put a stitch on the artery	A veces el cirujano necesitará coger un punto en la arteria	(ah veh-sees ehl see-roo-**hah**-noh neh-seh-see-tahr-**ah** koh-hehr oon **poon**-toh ehn lah ahr-tehr-**ee**-ah)
12. The needle can also cause an abnormal connection between the artery and vein by the hip	También, la aguja puede causar una conexión anormal entre la arteria y la vena	(tahm-bee-**ehn**, lah ah-**goo**-hah poo-**eh**-deh kah-oo-**sahr** oon-ah koh-nehk-see-**ohn** ah-nohr-**mahl** ehn-treh lah ahr-tehr-**ee**-ah ee lah **veh**-nah)
13. This is called an arteriovenous fistula	Esto se llama una fistula arteriovenosa	(ehs-toh seh **yah**-mah oon-ah fees-**too**-lah ahr-tehr-ee-oh-veh-**noh**-sah)

14.	Sometimes they heal on their own without treatment	A veces se curan por si mismas sin tratamiento	(ah veh-sehs seh **koo**-rahn-pohr see **mees**-mahs seen trah-tah-mee-**ehn**-toh)
15.	Sometimes the surgeon will need to put a stitch on the artery	A veces el cirujano necesitará coger un punto en la arteria	(ah veh-sehs ehl see-roo-**hah**-noh neh-seh-see-tahr-**ah** koh-**hehr** oon **poon**-toh ehn lah ahr-tehr-**ee**-ah)
16.	This is very rare	Esto es muy raro	(**ehs**-toh ehs moo-ee **rahr**-oh)
17.	Do you understand?	¿Entiende?	(ehn-tee-**ehn**-deh)
18.	Do you have any questions?	¿Tiene alguna pregunta?	(tee-**ehn**-eh ahl-**goon**-ah preh-**goon**-tah)
19.	Please read this	Por favor lea esto	(pohr fah-**vohr leh**-ah ehs-toh)
20.	We need your written consent	Necesitamos su firma de consentimiento	(neh-seh-see-**tah**-mohs soo **feer**-mah deh kohn-sehn-tee-mee-**ehn**-toh)
21.	Sign here	Firme aquí	(**feer**-meh ah-**kee**)

IMAGING GUIDED PROCEDURES

3. ARTERIOGRAPHY INSTRUCTIONS DURING PROCEDURE

1.	I need to check your pulse	Necesito chequear su pulso	(neh-seh-**see**-toh cheh-keh-**ahr** soo **pool**-soh)
2.	You will feel some pressure	Sentirá alguna presión	(sehn-teer-**ah** ahl-**goon**-ah preh-see-**ohn**)
3.	We need to shave this area to avoid infection	Necesitamos afeitar esta área para evitar infección	(neh-seh-see-**tah**-mohs ah-feh-ee-**tahr** ehs-tah **ah**-reh-ah pah-rah eh-vee-**tahr** een-fehk-see-**ohn**)

4.	This is antiseptic	Esto es un antiséptico	(ehs-toh ehs oon ahn-tee-**sehp**-tee-koh)
5.	Cold and wet	Frío y húmedo	(**free**-oh ee **oo**-mee-doh)
6.	This is local anesthesia	Esto es anestesia local	(ehs-toh ehs ahn-ehs-tehs-**ee**-ah loh-**kahl**)
7.	A little stick and some burning	Un pinchazo pequeño y un poco de ardor	(oon peen-**chah**-soh peh-**keh**-nyoh ee oon **poh**-koh deh ahr-**dohr**)
8.	The worst part is over	La peor parte se terminó	(lah peh-**ohr** pahr-teh seh tehr-mee-**noh**)
9.	Also, we can give you medicine to prevent pain and nervousness	También podemos darle alguna medicina para evitar dolor y nerviosismo	(tahm-bee-**ehn** poh-**deh**-mohs dahr-leh ahl-**goon**-ah meh-dee-**see**-nah pah-rah eh-vee-**tahr** doh-**lohr** ee nehr-vee-oh **sees**-moh)
10.	Everything is going well	Todo va bien	(toh-doh vah bee-**ehn**)
11.	Take a deep breath and hold it	Respire profundamente y aguante	(reh-**spee**-reh proh-foon-dah-**mehn**-teh ee ah-goo-**ahn**-teh)
12.	Hold your breath	Aguante su respiración	(ah-goo-**ahn**-teh soo reh-spee-rah-see-**ohn**)
13.	Breathe	Respire	(reh-**spee**-reh)
14.	Do not move	No se mueva	(noh seh moo-**eh**-vah)
15.	We need to take more radiographs	Necesitamos tomar más radiografías	(neh-seh-see-**tah**-mohs toh-**mahr mahs** rah-dee-oh-grah-**fee**-ahs)
16.	You will feel hot when the contrast is injected	Sentirá algo caliente cuando le inyecte la tinta	(sehn-tee-**rah** ahl-goh kah-lee-**ehn**-teh koo-**ahn**-doh leh een-**yehk**-teh lah **teen**-tah)
17.	We are almost finished	Casi terminamos	(kah-see tehr-mee-**nah**-mohs)

4. ARTERIOGRAPHY POST PROCEDURE

1.	I am going to remove the catheter now	Voy a sacar el catéter ahora	(voy ah sah-**kahr** ehl kah-**teh**-tehr ah-**ohr**-ah)
2.	The catheter is out	El catéter está afuera	(ehl kah-**teh**-tehr ehs-**tah** ah-foo-**ehr**-ah)
3.	You need to stay in bed and keep your leg straight for 6 hours	Necesita quedarse en la cama sin mover las piernas por seis horas	(neh-seh-**see**-tah keh-**dahr**-seh ehn lah **kah**-mah seen moh-**vehr** lahs pee-**ehr**-nahs pohr seh-ees **ohr**-ahs)
4.	If bleeding occurs in the wound, apply direct pressure and call the nurse	Si tiene sangramiento en la herida aplique presión y llame a la enfermera	(see tee-**ehn**-eh sahn-grah-mee-**ehn**-toh ehn lah ehr-**ee**-dah ah-plee-keh preh-see-**ohn** ee **yah**-meh ah lah ehn-fehr **mehr**-ah)
5.	You can eat when you get upstairs to your room	Puede comer cuando regrese a la habitación	(poo-**eh**-deh koh-**mehr** koo-**ahn**-doh reh-**greh**-seh ah lah ah-bee-tah-see-**ohn**)
6.	Someone will come and bring you to your room	Alguien vendrá y le llevará a su habitación	(ahl-goo-**ee**-ehn vehn-**drah** ee leh yeh-vahr-**ah** ah soo ah-bee-tah-see-**ohn**)

5. CEREBRAL ARTERIOGRAM

1.	You are here for an arteriogram of the brain	Usted está aquí para un arteriograma del cerebro	(oos-tehd ehs-**tah** ah-**kee** pah-rah oon ahr-tehr-ee-oh-**grah**-mah dehl sehr-**eh**-broh)

2. The ultrasound shows narrowing of the arteries that go to the brain	El ultrasonido demuestra estrechez en las arterias que van al cerebro	(ehl ool-trah-sohn-**ee**-doh deh-moo-**ehs**-trah ehs-treh-**chehs** ehn lahs ahr-tehr-**ee**-ahs keh vahn ahl sehr-**eh**-broh)
3. Carotid stenosis	Estenosis carótida	(ehs-tehn-**oh**-sees kah-**roh**-tee-dah)
4. This may increase your risk for a stroke	Esto puede aumentar el riesgo de un derrame cerebral	(ehs-toh poo-**eh**-deh ah-oo-mehn-**tahr** ehl ree-**ehs**-goh deh oon dehr-**ah**-meh sehr-eh-**brahl**)
5. This test, an arteriogram, gives a more detailed and accurate picture than U/S	Este arteriograma nos da una radiografía con más detalles y precisión que el ultrasonidó	(ehs-teh ahr-tehr-ee-oh-**grah**-mah nohs dah oon-ah rah-dee-oh-grah-**fee**-ah kohn **mahs** deh-**tah**-yehs ee preh-see-see-**ohn** keh ehl ool-trah-soh-nee-**doh**)
6. Your doctor asked us to do this test to check for narrowing in the arteries that go to the brain	Su doctor solicitó esta prueba para chequear la estrechez de las arterias	(soo dohk-**tohr** soh-lee-see-**toh** ehs-tah proo-**eh**-bah pah-rah cheh-keh-**ahr** lah ehs-treh-**chehs** deh lahs ahr-tehr-**ee**-ahs)
7. The results will help determine which treatment is best for you	Los resultados ayudarán a determinar el mejor tratamiento por usted	(lohs reh-sool-**tah**-dohs eye-oo-dahr-**ahn** ah deh-tehr-mee-**nahr** ehl meh-**hohr** trah-tah-mee-**ehn**-toh pohr oos-**tehd**)
8. Do you have or have you had numbness in your arm or leg?	¿Tiene o ha tenido su brazo o pierna adormecida?	(tee-**ehn**-eh oh ah teh-**nee**-doh soo **brah**-soh oh pee-**ehr**-nah ah-dohr-meh-**see**-dah)
9. Do you have dizziness?	¿Tiene mareos?	(tee-**ehn**-eh mahr-**eh**-ohs)
10. You had an abnormal CT scan of the brain	La tomografía computarizada del cerebro es anormal	(lah toh-moh-grah-**fee**-ah kohm-poo-tahr-ee-**sah**-dah dehl sehr-**eh**-broh ehs ah-nohr-**mahl**)
11. There was some bleeding in the brain	Usted tuvo una hemorragia en el cerebro	(oos-tehd **too**-voh oon-ah eh-mahr-ah-**hee**-ah ehn ehl sehr-**eh**-broh)

12. The most common cause of this bleeding is an aneurysm	La causa más común de esta hemorragia es un aneurisma	(lah kah-**oo**-sah **mahs** koh-**moon** deh ehs-tah eh-mohr-ah-**hee**-ah ehs oon ahn-eh-oo-**rees**-mah)
13. The purpose ot this test is to check for an aneurysm	El propósito de esta prueba es chequear si hay un aneurisma	(ehl proh-**poh**-see-toh deh ehs-tah proo-**eh**-bah ehs cheh-keh-**ahr** see eye oon ahn-eh-oo-**rees**-mah)
14. We need to determine the site of bleeding	Necesitamos determinar el lugar de la hemorragia	(neh-seh-see-**tah**-mohs deh-tehr-mee-**nahr** ehl loo-**gahr** deh lah ehm-ohr-ah-**hee**-ah)
15. This will help to make the surgery easier for the surgeons	Esto ayudará a hacer la cirugía más fácil para el cirujano	(ehs-toh eye-oo-dahr-**ah** ah ah-**sehr** lah see-roo-**hee**-ah **mahs fah**-seel pah-rah ehl see-roo-**hah**-noh)
16. You have a brain tumor	Usted tiene un tumor en el cerebro	(oos-tehd tee-**ehn**-eh oon too-**mohr** ehn ehl sehr-**eh**-broh)
17. The purpose of this test is to determine	El propósito de esta prueba es determinar	(ehl proh-**poh**-see-toh deh ehs-tah proo-**eh**-bah ehs deh-tehr-mee-**nahr**)
18. Which blood vessels go to the tumor	Cuales vasos sanguíneos van al tumor	(koo-**ahl**-ehs vah-sohs sahn-goo-**ee**-neh-ohs vahn ahl too-**mohr**)
19. This information is important to the surgeons who will remove the tumor	Esta información es importante para el cirujano quien removerá el tumor	(ehs-tah een-fohrmah-see-**ohn** ehs eem-pohr-**tahn**-teh pah-rah ehl see-roo-**hah**-noh kee-ehn reh-moh-vehr-**ah** ehl too-**mohr**)
20. In addition, we may block one of the arteries by injecting clotting material	Además, podemos bloquear algúnas de las arterias cuando inyectamos material de coágulos	(ah-deh-**mahs**, poh-deh-mohs bloh-keh-**ahr** ahl-**goo**-nahs deh lahs ahr-tehr-**ee**-ahs koo-**ahn**-doh een-yehk-**tah**-mohs mah-tehr-ee-**ahl** deh koh-**ah**-goo-lohs)

21.	This will help to decrease the risk of bleeding during surgery	Esto ayudará a reducir el riesgo de hemorragia durante la cirugía	(ehs-toh eye-oo-dahr-**ah** ah reh-doo-**seer** ehl ree-**ehs**-goh deh ehm-oh-rah-**hee**-ah doo-**rahn**-teh lah see-roo-**hee**-ah)
22.	Particles	Partículas	(pahr-**tee**-koo-lahs)
23.	Coils	Espirales metálicos	(ehs-peer-**ahl**-ehs meh-**tahl**-ee-kohs)
24.	The purpose of this test is to check for an abnormal communication	El propósito de esta prueba es chequear si hay una communicación anormal	(ehl proh-**poh**-see-toh deh ehs-tah proo-**eh**-bah ehs cheh-keh-**ahr** see eye oon-ah koh-moon-ee-kah-see-**ohn** ah-nohr-**mahl**)
25.	Between the arteries and veins in the brain	Entre las arterias y venas en el cerebro	(ehn-treh lahs ahr-ter-**ee**-ahs ee vehn-ahs ehn ehl sehr-**eh**-broh)
26.	AVM	Malformación arteriovenosa	(mahl-fohr-mah-see-**ohn** ahr-tehr-ee-oh-vehn-**oh**-sah)
27.	AVF	Fístula arteriovenosa	(**fees**-too-lah ahr-tehr-ee-oh-vehn-**oh**-sah)
28.	Epistaxis	Sangrando por la nariz	(sahn-**grahn**-doh pohr lah nah-**rees**)
29.	Trauma to the neck	Trauma del cuello	(trah-**oo**-mah dehl koo-**eh**-loh)
30.	Bullet	Bala	(**bah**-lah)
31.	Knife	Cuchillo	(koo-**chee**-yoh)
32.	The purpose of this test is to check for an injury	El propósito de esta prueba es para chequear por areas dañadas	(ehl proh-**poh**-see-toh deh ehs-tah proo-**eh**-bah ehs pah-rah cheh-keh-**ahr** pohr ahr-**eh**-ahs deh-**nyah**-dahs)
33.	To the arteries which go to your brain and arms	De las arterias que van al cerebro y a los brazos	(deh lahs ahr-tehr-**ee**-ahs keh vahn ahl sehr-**eh**-broh ee ah lohs **brah**-sohs)

6. PULMONARY ARTERIOGRAM

1. The purpose of this test	El propósito de esta prueba	(ehl proh-**poh**-see-toh deh ehs-tah proo-**eh**-bah)
2. Is to check for a blood clot in the lungs	Es para chequear si hay algún coágulo de sangre en los pulmones	(ehs pah-rah cheh-keh-**ahr** see ey ahl-**goon** koh-**ah**-goo-loh deh **sahn**-greh ehn lohs pool-**mohn**-ehs)
3. This is a very serious disease	Esta es una enfermedad muy seria	(ehs-tah ehs oon-ah ehn-fehr-mee-**dahd** moo-ee sehr-**ee**-ah)
4. It can kill a person	Puede matar a una persona	(poo-**eh**-deh mah-**tahr** ah oon-ah pehr-**sohn**-ah)
5. During this procedure	Durante este procedimiento	(doo-**rahn**-teh ehs-teh proh-see-dee-mee-**ehn**-toh)
6. It is possible that the heart may develop an abnormal rhythm	Es posible que el corazón puede a desarrollar un ritmo anormal	(ehs poh-**see**-bleh keh ehl kohr-ah-**sohn** poo-**eh**-deh ah dehs-ah-roh-**yahr** oon **reet**-moh ah-nohr-**mahl**)
7. Almost always this is temporary and not significant	Casi siempre esto es transitorio y no es significativo	(kah-see see-**ehm**-preh ehs-toh ehs trahn-see-tohr-**ee**-oh ee noh ehs seeg-nee-fee-kah-**tee**-voh)
8. However, it is possible that we may need to give you medicines for your heart	Sin embargo es posible que necesitemos darle alguna medicina para su corazón	(seen ehm-**bahr**-goh ehs poh-**see**-bleh keh neh-seh-see-**teh**-mohs dahr-le ahl-**goo**-nah meh-dee-**see**-nah pah-rah soo kohr-ah-**sohn**)
9. Or even an electric shock to help it beat correctly and restore the normal rhythm	O darle una sacudida eléctrica para restablecer el ritmo normal	(oh **dahr**-leh oon-ah sah-koo-**dee**-dah eh-**lehk**-tree-koh pah-rah reh-stah-bleh-**sehr** ehl **reet**-moh nohr-**mahl**)

7. BIOPSY

1. You are here for a biopsy of the liver	Usted esta aquí para una biopsia del hígado	(oos-tehd ehs-tah ah-**kee** pah-rah oon-ah bee-ohp-**see**-ah dehl **ee**-gah-doh)
2. The purpose of this test is to find out if you have a tumor	El propósito de esta prueba es ver si usted tiene un tumor	(ehl proh-**poh**-see-toh deh ehs-tah proo-**eh**-bah ehs vehr see oos-**tehd** tee-**ehn**-eh oon too-**mohr**)
3. And if it is a tumor	Y si es un tumor	(ee see ehs oon too-**mohr**)
4. To determine if it is benign or malignant	determinar si es benigno o maligno	(deh-tehr-mee-**nahr** see ehs beh-**neeg**-noh oh mah-**leeg**-noh)
5. We will use U/S to guide the needle	Usaremos el ultrasonido para guiar la aguja	(oo-sahr-**eh**-mohs ehl ool-trah-soh-**nee**-doh pah-rah goo-ee-**ahr** lah ah-**goo**-hah)
6. We will use the CT scanner to guide the needle	Usaremos la máquina de tomografía computarizada para guiar la aguja	(oo-sahr-**eh**-mohs lah **mah**-kee-nah deh toh-mah-grah-**fee**-ah kohm-poo-tahr-ee-**sah**-dah pah-rah goo-ee-**ahr** lah ah-**goo**-hah)
7. The main risk is bleeding	El riesgo principal es hemorragia	(ehl ree-**ehs**-goh preen-see-**pahl** ehs eh-mohr-ah-**hee**-ah)
8. Usually this is not significant	Usualmente no es significativo	(oo-soo-ahl-**mehn**-teh noh ehs seeg-nee-fee-kah-**tee**-voh)

8. CORONARY ARTERIOGRAM

1. The purpose of this test	El propósito de esta prueba	(ehl proh-**poh**-see-toh deh ehs-tah proo-**eh**-bah)

2. Is to check for narrowing in the arteries of the heart	Es para chequear por estrechez de las arterias del corazón	(ehs pah-rah cheh-keh-**ahr** pohr ehs-treh-**chehs** deh lahs ahr-tehr-**ee**-ahs dehl kohr-ah-**sohn**)

3. See section on Arteriography General Information

9. IVC FILTER

1. The purpose of this procedure	El propósito de esta prueba	(ehl proh-**poh**-see-toh deh ehs-tah proo-**eh**-bah)
2. Is to protect your lungs from blood clots	Es proteger sus pulmones de coágulos de sangre	(ehs proh-teh-**hehr** soos pool-**mohn**-ehs deh koh-**ah**-goo-lohs deh **sahn**-greh)
3. Which may break off from veins in your legs and go to the lungs	Los cuales pueden separarse de las venas en sus piernas e irse a los pulmones	(lohs koo-**ahl**-ehs poo-**eh**-dehn seh-pahr-**ahr**-seh deh lahs veh-nahs ehn soos pee-**ehr**-nahs eh **eer**-seh ah lohs pool-**mohn**-ehs)
4. For this procedure we will put a catheter into the large vein in the neck	Para este procedimiento pondremos un catéter dentro de la vena grande en el cuello	(pah-rah ehs-teh proh-see-dee-mee-**ehn**-toh pohn-**dreh**-mohs oon kah-**teh**-tehr dehn-troh deh lah **veh**-nah **grahn**-deh ehn ehl koo-**eh**-yoh)
5. Internal jugular vein	La vena yugular interna	(lah **veh**-nah yoo-goo-**lahr** een-**tehr**-nah)
6. We will then position the catheter in the inferior vena cava (IVC)	Entonces colocaremos el catéter en la vena cava inferior	(ehn-**tohn**-sehs koh-loh-kahr-**eh**-mohs ehl kah-**teh**-tehr ehn lah **vehn**-ah **kah**-vah een-tehr-ee-**ohr**)
7. Below the renal veins	Debajo de las venas renales	(deh-**bah**-hoh deh lahs **veh**-nahs reh-**nahl**-ehs)

8. Then we will place/put a filter into the IVC	Entonces pondremos el filtro dentro de la vena cava inferior	(ehn-**tohn**-sehs pohn-**dreh**-mohs ehl **feel**-troh dehn-troh deh lah **veh**-nah **kah**-vah een-fehr-ee-**ohr**)
9. Usually this procedure is helpful	Usualmente este procedimiento es útil	(oo-soo-ahl-**mehn**-teh ehs-teh proh-seh-dee-mee-**ehn**-toh ehs **oo**-teel)
10. However, sometimes a person can get a blood clot in the lungs	Sin embargo, a veces una persona puede tener un coágulo en los pulmones	(seen ehm-**bahr**-goh ah **veh**-sehs oon-ah pehr-**sohn**-ah poo-**eh**-deh tehn-**ehr** oon koh-**ah**-goo-loh)
11. This occurs in less than 5%	Esto ocurre en menos de un cinco por ciento	(ehs-toh oh-**koo**-reh ehn **meh**-nohs deh oon **seen**-koh pohr see-**ehn**-toh)

10. MYELOGRAM

1. You are here for a myelogram	Usted esta aquí para un mielograma	(oos-**tehd** ehs-tah ah-**kee** pah-rah oon mee-ehl-oh-**grah**-mah)
2. The purpose of this test	El propósito de esta prueba	(ehl proh-**poh**-see-toh deh ehs-tah proo-**eh**-bah)
3. Is to check for compression of the spinal cord and nerves	Es para chequear la compresión de la médula espinal y los nervios	(ehs pah-rah cheh-keh-**ahr** lah kohm-preh-see-**ohn** deh lah **meh**-doo-lah ehs-pee-**nahl** ee lohs nehr-**vee**-ohs)
4. We will put a needle	Pondremos una aguja	(pohn-**dreh**-mohs oon-ah ah-**goo**-hah)

5. Into the space around the spinal cord and inject contrast	Dentro del espacio alrededor de la médula espinal e inyectare tinta	(dehn-troh dehl ehs-pah-**see**-oh ahl-reh-deh-**dohr** deh lah **meh**-doo-lah ehs-pee-**nahl** eh een-yehk-**tahr**-eh **teen**-tah)
6. The table will move/tilt up and down	La mesa se moverá hacía arriba y abajo	(lah **meh**-sah seh moh-vehr-**ah** ah-**see**-ah ah-**ree**-bah ee ah-**bah**-hoh)
7. Then we will take x-rays	Entonces tomaremos radiografías	(ehn-**tohn**-sehs toh-mahr-**eh**-mohs rah-dee-oh-grah-**fee**-ahs)
8. After the x-rays are completed	Después que se completen las radiografías	(dehs-poo-**ehs** keh seh kohm-pleh-**tehn** lahs rah-dee-oh-grah-**fee**-ahs)
9. You will have a CT scan	Usted tendrá una tomografía computada	(oos-**tehd** tehn-**drah** oon-ah toh-moh-grah-**fee**-ah kohm-poo-**tah**-dah)
10. The x-ray dye in the space around the spinal cord	La tinta dentro del espacio alrededor de la médula espinal	(lah **teen**-tah dehn-troh dehl eh-spah-**see**-oh ahl-reh-deh-**dohr** deh lah **meh**-doo-lah ehs-pee-**nahl**)
11. Produces a more detailed CT scan	Produce una tomografía computada más detallada	(proh-**doo**-seh oon-ah toh-moh-grah-**fee**-ah kohm-poo-**tah**-dah **mahs** deh-tah-**yah**-dah)

11. PERCUTANEOUS ABSCESS DRAINAGE (PAD)

1. You have an abscess in your pelvis	Tiene un absceso en la pelvis	(tee-**ehn**-eh oon ahb-**seh**-soh ehn lah **pehl**-vees)
2. The purpose of this test	El propósito de esta prueba	(ehl proh-**poh**-see-toh deh ehs-tah proo-**eh**-bah)

3. Is to drain the abscess with a tube	Es drenar el absceso con un tubo	(ehs dreh-**nahr** ehl ahb-**seh**-soh kohn oon **too**-boh)
4. Usually this treatment is effective	Usualmente este tratamiento es efectivo	(oos-oo-ahl-**mehn**-teh ehs-teh trah-tah-mee-**ehn**-toh ehs eh-fehk-**tee**-voh)
5. And surgery can be avoided	Y se puede evitar la cirugía	(ee seh poo-**eh**-deh eh-vee-**tahr** lah see-roo-**hee**-ah)
6. The tube will need to stay in anywhere from 2 days to 2 weeks	El tubo necesita quedarse adentro por dos días a dos semanas	(ehl **too**-boh neh-seh-**see**-tah keh-**dahr**-seh ah-**dehn**-troh pohr dohs **dee**-ahs ah dohs seh-**mah**-nahs)

12. PERCUTANEOUS NEPHROSTOMY

1. The drainage of your kidney is blocked	El drenaje de su riñón está bloqueado	(ehl dreh-**nah**-heh deh soo ree-**nyohn** ehs-**tah** bloh-keh-**ah**-doh)
2. The purpose of this test	El propósito de esta prueba	(ehl proh-**poh**-see-toh deh ehs-tah proo-**eh**-bah)
3. Is to drain the kidney in a tube	Es drenar el riñón con un tubo	(ehs dreh-**nahr** ehl ree-**nyohn** kohn oon **too**-boh)
4. This can help prevent infection	Esto puede ayudar a evitar infección	(ehs-toh poo-**eh**-deh eye-oo-**dahr** ah eh-vee-**tahr** ehn-fehk-see-**ohn**)
5. And loss of function of the kidney	Y la pérdida de función del riñón	(ee lah **pehr**-dee-dah deh foon-see-**ohn** dehl ree-**nyohn**)

13. PERCUTANEOUS TRANSLUMINAL ANGIOPLASTY

1. You have an area of narrowing in the artery	Usted tiene una área estrecha en la arteria	(oos-**tehd** tee-**eh**-neh oon-ah **ahr**-eh-ah ehs-**treh**-chah ehn lah ahr-tehr-**ee**-ah)
2. The purpose of angioplasty	El propósito de la angioplastia	(ehl proh-**poh**-see-toh deh lah ahn-hee-oh-plahs-**tee**-ah)
3. Is to increase blood flow to the artery	Es aumentar el flujo en la arteria	(ehs ah-oo-mehn-**tahr** ehl **floo**-hoh ehn lah ahr-tehr-**ee**-ah)
4. A balloon in inflated in the area of narrowing	Un globo es instalado en el área estrecha	(oon **gloh**-boh ehs eens-tah-**lah**-doh ehn ehl **ahr**-eh-ah eh-**streh**-cha)
5. Usually this is an effective treatment	Usualmente este es un tratamiento efectivo	(oos-oo-ahl-**mehn**-teh ehs-teh ehs oon trah-tah-mee-**ehn**-toh eh-fehk-**tee**-voh)
6. The artery remains open in 60% after 5 years	La arteria permanece abierta en un sesenta por ciento después de cinco años	(lah ahr-tehr-**ee**-ah pehr-mahn-**eh**-seh ah-bee-**ehr**-tah ehn oon seh-**sehn**-tah pohr see-**ehn**-toh dehs-poo-**ehs** deh **seen**-koh **ah**-nyohs)
7. In about 1% of persons	En cerca de uno por ciento de las personas	(enh **sehr**-kah deh oon-ah pohr see-**ehn**-toh deh lahs pehr-**sohn**-ahs)
8. The artery may rupture/ break	La arteria puede romperse	(lah ahr-tehr-**ee**-ah poo-**eh**-deh rohm-**pehr**-seh)
9. And you may need surgery to repair the artery	Y usted podrá necesitar cirugía para reparar la arteria	(ee oos-tehd poh-**drah** neh-seh-see-**tahr** see-roo-**hee**-ah pah-rah reh-pahr-**ahr** lah ahr-tehr-**ee**-ah)

14. PERIPHERALLY INSERTED CENTRAL CATHETER (PICC) LINE

1. This is a special type of IV	Este es un tipo especial de línea intravenosa	(ehs-teh ehs oon **tee**-poh ehs-peh-see-**ahl** deh **leen**-eh-ah een-trah-vehn-**oh**-sah)
2. Sometimes it can function several weeks	A veces funciona por varias semanas	(ah **veh**-sehs foon-see-**ohn**-ah\` pohr vahr-**ee**-ahs seh-**mahn**-ahs)
3. Do you want it put into your right arm?	¿La quiere en el brazo derecho?	(lah kee-**ehr**-eh ehn ehl **brah**-soh deh-**reh**-choh)
4. Or left arm?	¿O en el brazo izquierdo?	(oh ehn ehl **brah**-soh ees-kee-**ehr**-doh)

15. STENT PLACEMENT

1. This procedure is similar to angioplasty	Este procedimiento es parecido a la angioplastia	(ehs-teh proh-seh-dee-mee-**ehn**-toh ehs pahr-eh-**see**-doh ah lah ahn-hee-oh-plahs-**tee**-ah)
2. However, in addition to using a balloon	Sin embargo además de usar un globo	(seen ehm-**bahr**-goh ah-deh-**mahs** deh oo-**sahr** oon **gloh**-boh)
3. A metal bridge is put into the artery	Un puente metálico se pone dentro de la arteria	(oon poo-**ehn**-teh meh-**tahl**-ee-koh seh poh-neh dehn-troh deh lah ahr-tehr-**ee**-ah)

4. This will remain in the artery forever	Este se quedará en la arteria para siempre	(ehs-teh seh keh-dahr-**ah** ehn lah ahr-tehr-**ee**-ah pah-rah see-**ehm**-preh)
5. Usually it lasts longer than angioplasty	Usualmente dura más que la angioplastia	(oos-oo-ahl-**mehn**-teh doo-rah **mahs** keh lah ahn-hee-oh-plahs-**tee**-ah)

16. THROMBOLYSIS

1. You have a blood clot in the arteries of your leg	Usted tiene un coágulo en la arteria de su pierna	(oos-**tehd** tee-**ehn**-eh oon koh-**ah**-goo-loh ehn lah ahr-tehr-**ee**-ah deh soo pee-**ehr**-nah)
2. The purpose of this procedure is to dissolve the blood clot	El propósito de este procedimiento es disolver los coágulos	(ehl proh-**poh**-see-toh deh ehs-teh proh-seh-dee-mee-**ehn**-toh ehs dee-sohl-**vehr** los koo-**ah**-goo-lohs)
3. We will give you clot dissolving medicine	Le daremos medicina para disolver los coágulos	(leh dahr-**eh**-mohs meh-dee-**see**-nah pah-rah dee-sohl-**vehr** lohs koh-**ah**-goo-lohs)
4. Thru a catheter placed in the clot	A travez de un catéter colocado en el coágulo	(ah-trah-**vehs** deh oon kah-**teh**-tehr koh-loh-**kah**-doh ehn ehl koh-**ah**-goo-loh)
5. After the clot is dissolved you may still need to have angioplasty or surgery	Después de este procedimiento puede que todavía necesite angioplastia o cirugía	(dehs-poo-**ehs** deh eh-steh proh-seh-dee-mee-**ehn**-toh poo-**eh**-deh keh toh-dah-**vee**-ah neh-seh-**see**-teh ahn-hee-oh-plahs-**tee**-ah oh see-roo-**hee**-ah)
6. The main risk is bleeding	El riesgo principal es hemorragia	(ehl ree-**ehs**-goh preen-see-**pahl** ehs ehm-ohr-ah-**hee**-ah)

7. About 1% of persons will have bleeding in their abdomen or brain	Cerca de uno por ciento de las personas tendrán hemorragia en el abdomen o el cerebro	(**sehr**-kah deh oon-oh pohr see-**ehn**-toh deh lahs pehr-**soh**-nahs tehn-**drahn** ehm-ohr-ah-**hee**-ah ehn ehl ahb-**doh**-mehn oh ehl sehr-**eh**-broh)
8. Sometimes the clot cannot be dissolved	A veces el coágulo no se puede disolver	(ah **veh**-sehs ehl koh-**ah**-goo-loh noh seh poo-**eh**-deh dee-sohl-**vehr**)
9. You may need emergency surgery	Usted puede necesitar cirugía de emergencia	(oos-**tehd** poo-**eh**-deh neh-seh-see-**tahr** seer-oo-**hee**-ah deh eh-mehr-hehn-**see**-ah)

17. VENOGRAM

1. The purpose of this test	El propósito de esta prueba	(ehl proh-**poh**-see-toh deh ehs-tah proo-**eh**-bah)
2. Is to check for a blood clot in your legs	Es para chequear por un coágulo en sus piernas	(ehs pah-rah cheh-keh-**ahr** pohr oon koh-**ah**-goo-loh ehn soos pee-**ehr**-nahs)
3. I will put an IV in your foot	Le pondré una línea intravenosa en su pie	(leh pohn-**dreh** oon-ah **lee**-neh-ah een-trah-vehn-**oh**-sah ehn soo **pee**-eh)
4. And then inject contrast	Y entonces inyectaré tinta	(ee ehn-**tohn**-sehs een-yehk-tahr-**eh** teen-tah)
5. Then we will take x-rays	Entonces le tomaremos rayos-equis	(ehn-**tohn**-sehs leh toh-mahr-**eh**-mohs **reye**-ohs **eh**-kees)

INFORMED CONSENT

Section Eight

1.	The risks of this procedure are	Los riesgos de este procedimiento son	(lohs ree-**ehs**-gohs deh ehs-teh proh-see-dee-mee-**ehn**-toh sohn)
2.	1 out of 10	Uno de diez	(**oon**-on deh **dee**-ehs)
3.	1 out of 100	Uno de cien	(**oon**-oh deh **see**-ehn)
4.	1 out of 1,000	Uno de mil	(**oon**-oh deh **meel**)
5.	Bleeding	Hemorragia	(ehm-ohr-ah **hee** ah)
6.	Infection	Infección	(een-fehk-see-**ohn**)
7.	Seizure	Convulsión	(kohn-vool-see-**ohn**)
8.	Stroke	Derrame cerebral	(deh-**rah**-meh seh-rah-**brahl**)
9.	Heart attack	Ataque al corazón	(ah-**tah**-keh ahl kohr-ah-**sohn**)
10.	Arrhythmia	Ritmo anormal del corazón	(**reet**-moh ah-nohr-**mahl** dehl kohr-ah-**sohn**)
11.	Lack of improvement in your condition	Falta de mejoría en su condición	(**fahl**-tah deh meh-hohr-**ee**-ah ehn soo kohn-dee-see-**ohn**)
12.	Blood transfusion	Transfusión de sangre	(trahns-foo-see-**ohn** deh **sahn**-greh)
13.	All of the blood is screened for HIV and hepatitis	Toda la sangre se ha analizado por SIDA y hepatitis	(**toh**-dah lah **sahn**-greh seh ah ahn-ah-lee-**sah**-doh pohr **see**-dah ee eh-pah-**tee**-tees)
14.	Do you understand?	¿Entiende?	(ehn-tee-**ehn**-deh)
15.	Do you have any questions?	¿Tiene algunas preguntas?	(tee-**ehn**-eh ahl-**goon**-ahs preh-**goon**-tahs)
16.	We need your written consent	Necesitamos su consentimiento de firma	(neh-seh-see-**tah**-mohs soo kohn-sehn-tee-mee-**ehn**-toh deh **feer**-mah)
17.	The form says that we have discussed the procedure with you	Este forma indica que hemos discutido el procedimiento con usted	(ehs-teh **fohr**-mah een-**dee**-kah keh **eh**-mohs dees-koo-**tee**-doh ehl proh-seh-dee-mee-**ehn**-toh kohn oos-**tehd**)

18.	Including the possible benefits, risks	Incluyendo la posibilidad de beneficios, riesgos	(een-kloo-**yehn**-doh lah poh-see-beel-ee-**dahd** deh behn-eh-fee-**see**-ohs ree-**ehs**-gohs)
19.	And alternative tests or treatments	Y pruebas alternativas	(ee proo-**eh**-bahs ahl-tehr-nah-**tee**-vahs)
20.	Also, that we have answered any questions you might have	También, indica que hemos contestado sus preguntas	(tahm-bee-**ehn**, een-**dee**-kah keh **eh**-mohs kohn-tehs-**tah**-doh soos preh-**goon**-tahs)
21.	Do you understand?	¿Entiende?	(ehn-tee-**ehn**-deh)
22.	Sign here	Firme aquí	(**feer**-meh ah-**kee**)

Disclaimer: Please note this section is only an introduction to the detailed topic of informed consent and does not in any way in and of itself constitute an adequate means of obtaining informed consent.

Section Nine

ADDITIONAL CLINICAL SPECIALITIES

1. OBSTETRICS

CHAPTER OUTLINE

AGE

1. How old are you?	¿Cuántos años tiene usted?	(koo-**ahn**-tohs **ahn**-yohs tee-**ehn**-eh oos-**tehd**)

GRAVITY AND PARITY (GP)

1. How many times have you been pregnant?	¿Cuántas veces ha estado embarazada?	(koo-**ahn**-tahs veh-sehs ah ehs-**tah**-doh ehm-bah-rah-**sah**-dah)
2. How many children do you have?	¿Cuántos hijos tiene?	(koo-**ahn**-tohs ee-hohs tee-**ehn**-eh)

3. How many were born full term (nine months)?	¿Cuántos nacieron en el tiempo correcto (nueve meses)?	(koo-**ahn**-tohs nah-see-**ehr**-ohn ehn ehl tee-**ehm**-poh koh-**rehk**-toh noo-**eh**-veh **meh**-sehs)
4. How many were born premature?	¿Cuántos nacieron prematuros?	(koo-**ahn**-tohs nah-see-**ehr**-ohn pree-mah-**toor**-ohs)
5. Have you had any miscarriages or abortions?	¿Ha tenido algunos abortos espontáneos o provocados?	(ah teh-**nee**-doh ahl-**goon**-ohs ah-**bohr**-tohs ehs-pohn-**tahn**-eh-oh oh proh-voh-**kah**-dohs)

LMP

1. When was your last normal menstrual period?	¿Cuándo fue su última regla normal?	(koo-**ahn**-doh foo-eh soo **ool**-tee-mah **reh**-glah nohr-**mahl**)
2. Was that the first day of your menstrual period?	¿Fue este el primer día de su última regla?	(foo-eh ehs-teh ehl pree-**mehr** **dee**-ah deh soo **ool**-tee-mah **reh**-glah)
3. Does your period come every month?	¿Le viene cada mes?	(leh vee-**ehn**-eh **kah**-dah mehs)
4. Were you taking birth control pills?	¿Tomó usted píldoras contraceptivas?	(toh-**moh** oos-tehd **peel**-dohr--ahs kohn-trah-sehp-**tee**-vahs)

EDC

1. When is your due date?	¿Cuál es la fecha esperada del nacimiento?	(koo-**ahl** ehs lah **feh**-chah ehs-pehr-**ah**-dah dehl nah-see-mee-**ehn**-toh)
2. Have you had an ultra-sound?	¿Ha tenido un ultrasonido?	(ah tehn-**ee**-doh oon ool-trah-sohn-**ee**-doh)
3. When?	¿Cuándo?	(koo-**ahn**-doh)
4. Where?	¿Dónde?	(**dohn**-deh)

5. Did the ultrasound change your due date?	¿El ultrasonido le cambió la fecha de naciemento?	(ehl ool-trah-sohn-**ee**-doh leh kahm-bee-**oh** lah **feh**-chah deh nah-see-mee-**ehn**-toh)

EGA

1. How many weeks have you been pregnant?	¿Cuántas semanas ha estado embarazada?	(koo-**ahn**-tahs seh-**mah**-nahs ah ehs-**tah**-doh ehm-bahr-ah-**sah**-dah)
2. You are 40 weeks pregnant	Usted tiene cuarenta semanas de embarazo	(oos-tehd tee-**ehn**-eh koo-ahr-**ehn**-tah seh-**mahn**-ahs deh ehm-bah-**rah**-soh)
3. How many months pregnant are you?	¿Cuántos meses ha estado embarazada?	(koo-**ahn**-tohs meh-sehs ah ehs-**tah**-doh ehm-bahr-ah-**sah**-dah)

UTERINE CONTRACTIONS

1. Are you having contractions?	¿Tiene contracciones?	(tee-**ehn**-eh kohn-trahk-see-**ohn**-ehs)
2. How frequently?	¿Con qué frecuencia?	(kohn **keh** freh-koo-ehn-**see**-ah)
3. How long do they last?	¿Cuánto tiempo duran?	(koo-**ahn**-toh tee-**ehm**-poh doo-rahn)
4. Are the pains strong?	¿Son fuertes los dolores?	(sohn foo-**ehr**-tehs lohs doh-**lohr**-ehs)
5. Please, point to where it hurts the most	Por favor enséñeme dónde le duele más	(pohr fah-**vohr** ehn-**seh**-nyeh-meh **dohn**-deh leh doo-**eh**-lah **mahs**)
6. In your abdomen?	¿En su abdomen?	(ehn soo ahb-**doh**-mehn)
7. In your back?	¿En su espalda?	(ehn soo ehs-**pahl**-dah)

8. In your back near the waist?	¿En su espalda cerca de la cintura?	(ehn soo ehs-**pahl**-dah **sehr**-kah deh lah seen-**too**-rah)
9. Since when have your contractions been regular and painful?	¿Desde cuándo tiene contracciones regulares y dolorosas?	(dehs-deh koo-**ahn**-doh tee-**ehn**-eh kohn-trahk-see-**ohn**-ehs reh-goo-**lahr**-ehs ee doh-lohr-**oh**-sahs)

BLEEDING

1. Have you had any vaginal bleeding?	¿Ha tenido sangramiento por la vagina?	(ah teh-**nee**-doh sahn-grah-mee-**ehn**-toh pohr lah vah-**hee**-nah)
2. A little or a lot?	¿Un poco o mucho?	(oon **poh**-koh oh **moo**-choh)
3. How many pads?	¿Cuántas toallas sanitarias?	(koo-**ahn**-tohs toh-**ah**-yahs sahn-ee-tahr-**ee**-ahs)
4. Was there any mucus mixed with the bleeding?	¿Algún moco en la sangre?	(ahl-**goon** moh-koh enh lah **sahn**-greh)

BAG OF WATER

1. Have you had leakage of water?	¿Ha tenido agua por la vagina?	(ah teh-**nee**-doh ah-**goo**-ah pohr lah vah-**hee**-nah)
2. A little or a lot?	¿Un poco o mucho?	(oon **poh**-koh oh **moo**-choh)
3. Has your bag of water ruptured?	¿Se le rompió la bolsa de agua?	(seh leh rohm-pee-**oh** lah **bohl**-sah deh ah-**goo**-ah)
4. When did it start leaking?	¿Cuándo comenzó?	(koo-**ahn**-doh koh-mehn-**soh**)
5. At what hour did it start?	¿A qué hora comenzó?	(ah **keh ohr**-ah koh-mehn-**soh**)
6. What color?	¿Qué color?	(**keh** koh-**lohr**)
7. Clear or dark?	¿Claro u oscuro?	(**klah**-roh oo ohs-**koo**-roh)
8. Speculum	Un espéculo	(oon ehs-**peh**-koo-loh)

FETAL MOVEMENT

1. Can you feel the baby moving?	¿Siente el bebé moverse?	(see-**ehn**-teh ehl beh-**beh** moh-**vehr**-seh)
2. When was the last time you felt the baby move?	¿Cuándo fue la última vez que sintió su bebé moverse?	(koo-**ahn**-doh foo-eh lah **ool**-tee-mah vehs keh seen-tee-**oh** soo beh-**beh** moh-**vehr**-seh)

WEIGHT GAIN

1. How much weight have you gained?	¿Cuánto ha aumentado de peso con este embarazo?	(koo-**ahn**-toh ah ah-oo-mehn-**tah**-doh deh **peh**-soh kohn ehs-teh ehm-bah-**rah**-soh)
2. How much did you weigh before this pregnancy?	¿Cuál fue su peso antes de este embarazo?	(koo-**ahl** foo-eh soo **peh**-soh ahn-tehs deh ehs-teh ehm-bah-**rah**-soh)
3. How much do you weigh now?	¿Cuál es su peso ahora?	(koo-**ahl** ehs soo **peh**-soh ah-**ohr**-ah)

PRENATAL CARE (PNC)

1. Have you had any PNC?	¿Ha tenido algún cuidado prenatal?	(ah teh-**nee**-doh ahl-**goon** koo-ee-**dah**-doh preh-nah-**tahl**)
2. Have you seen another doctor during this pregnancy?	¿Ha visitado algún doctor durante este embarazo?	(ah vee-see-**tah**-doh ahl-**goon** dohk-**tohr** doo-**rahn**-teh ehs-teh ehm-bah-**rah**-soh)
3. Where?	¿Dónde?	(**dohn**-deh)
4. When was your first visit to the doctor during this pregnancy?	¿Cuándo fue la primera cita con un doctor en este embarazo?	(koo-**ahn**-doh foo-eh lah pree-**meh**-rah **see**-tah kohn oon dohk-**tohr** ehn ehs-tah ehm-bah-**rah**-soh)
5. Have you had any problems with this pregnancy?	¿Ha tenido algunos problemas con este embarazo?	(ah teh-**nee**-doh ahl-**goo**-nohs proh-**bleh**-mahs kohn ehs-teh ehm-bah-**rah**-soh)

6. Have you had headaches or blurred vision?	¿Ha tenido dolores de cabeza o vista nublada?	(ah teh-**nee**-doh doh-**lohr**-ehs deh kah-**beh**-sah oh **vees**-tah noo-**blah**-dah)
7. Have you had high blood pressure?	¿Ha tenido la presión alta?	(ah teh-**nee**-doh lah preh-see-**ohn ahl**-tah)

PRENATAL LABS

1. Have you had any blood tests during this pregnancy?	¿Ha tenido algunas pruebas de sangre durante este embarazo?	(ah teh-**nee**-doh ahl-**goo**-nahs proo-**eh**-bahs deh **sahn**-greh doo-**rahn**-teh ehs-teh ehm-bah-**rah**-soh)
2. Blood type	Tipo de sangre	(**tee**-poh deh **sahn**-greh)
3. Syphilis	Sífilis	(**see**-fee-lees)
4. Rubella	Rubeola	(roo-beh-**oh**-lah)
5. Hepatitis	Hepatitis	(eh-pah-**tee**-tees)
6. Pap smear	Papanicolau	(pah-pah-nee-koh-**lah**-oo)
7. Hemoglobin	Hemoglobina	(ehm-oh-gloh-**bee**-nah)

OBSTETRIC HISTORY

1. How many children do you have?	¿Cuántos hijos tiene?	(koo-**ahn**-tohs **ee**-hohs tee-**ehn**-eh)
2. When was the first child born?	¿Cuándo nació el primer hijo?	(koo-**ahn**-doh nah-see-**oh** ehl pree-**mehr ee**-hoh)
3. The second?	¿El segundo?	(ehl seh-**goon**-doh)
4. The third?	¿El tercero?	(ehl tehr-**sehr**-oh)
5. The fourth?	¿El cuarto?	(ehl koo-**ahr**-toh)
6. Was it a boy or a girl?	¿Un niño o niña?	(oon **nee**-nyoh oh **nee**-nyah)
7. How much did the baby weigh?	¿Cuánto peso el bebé?	(koo-**ahn**-toh **peh**-soh ehl beh-**beh**)

8. What type of delivery?	¿Qué tipo de parto?	(**keh tee**-poh deh **pahr**-toh)
9. Vaginal or caesarean?	¿Vaginal o cesárea?	(vah-**hee**-nahl oh seh-**sahr**-eh-ah)
10. Why caesarean?	¿Por qué cesárea?	(pohr **keh** seh-**sahr**-eh-ah)
11. Did you have a long and difficult labor?	¿Tuvo un parto largo y difícil?	(**too**-voh oon **pahr**-toh **lahr**-goh ee dee-**fee**-seel)
12. How many hours?	¿Cuántas horas?	(koo-**ahn**-tohs **ohr**-ahs)
13. Where?	¿Dónde?	(**dohn**-deh)
14. At what hospital?	¿En qué hospital?	(ehn **keh** ohs-pee-**tahl**)
15. Were there any problems with the baby?	¿Algunos problemas con este bebé?	(ahl-**goon**-ohs proh-**bleh**-mahs kohn ehs-teh beh-**beh**)
16. Did you have any complications with your pregnancies?	¿Ha tenido complicaciones con los embarazos?	(ah teh-**nee**-doh kohm-plee-kah-see-**ohn**-ehs kohn lohs ehm-bahr-**ah**-sohs)
17. High blood pressure?	¿La presión alta?	(lah preh-see-**ohn ahl**-tah)
18. Hypertension?	¿Hipertensión?	(ee-pehr-rehn-see-**ohn**)
19. Excessive bleeding?	¿Sangramiento excesivo?	(sahn-grah-mee-**ehn**-toh ehx-seh-**see**-voh)

MENSTRUAL HISTORY

1. How old were you when your period started?	¿A qué edad le vino su regla por primera vez?	(ah **keh** eh-**dahd** leh **vee**-noh soo **reh**-glah pohr pree-**mehr**-ah-vehs)
2. How many weeks between periods?	¿Cuántas semanas entre los períodos menstruales?	(koo-**ahn**-tohs seh-**mahn**-ehs ehn-treh lohs pehr-**ee**-oh-dohs mehn-stroo-**ahl**-ehs)
3. How many days between periods?	¿Cuántos días entre los períodos?	(koo-**ahn**-tohs **dee**-ahs ehn-treh lohs pehr-**ee**-oh-dos)

4. How long does each period last?	¿Cuánto tiempo le dura la regla?	(koo-**ahn**-toh tee-**ehm**-poh leh **doo**-rah lah **reh**-glah)
5. Are the cycles regular?	¿Es su regla puntual?	(ehs soo **reh**-glah poon-too-**ahl**)
6. Pads	Toallas sanitarias	(toh-**ah**-yahs sahn-ee-tahr-**ee**-ahs)
7. Tampons	Tampones	(tahm-**pohn**-ehs)

GYNE HISTORY

1. Have you ever had an infection in your tubes?	¿Ha tenido algunas infecciones en sus trompas?	(ah teh-**nee**-doh ahl-**goon**-ahs een-fehk-see-**ohn**-ehs ehn soos **trohm**-pahs)
2. Were you hospitalized for that condition?	¿La internaron en el hospital por la infección?	(lah een-tehr-**nahr**-ohn ehn ehl ohs-pee-**tahl** pohr lah een-fehk-see-**ohn**)
3. Have you had any vaginal infection?	¿Ha tenido algunas infecciones vaginales?	(ah teh-**nee**-doh ahl-**goon**-ehs een-fehk-see-**ohn**-ehs vah-hee-**nahl**-ehs)
4. Herpes?	¿Herpes?	(**ehr**-pees)
5. Gonorrhea?	¿Gonorrea?	(goh-noh-**reh**-ah)
6. Syphilis?	¿Sífilis?	(**see**-fee-lees)
7. Condyloma, warts?	¿Condiloma verrugas?	kohn-dee-**loh**-mah veh-**roo**-gahs)
8. Have you had any vaginal discharge?	¿Ha tenido algún flujo por la vagina?	(ah teh-**nee**-doh ah-**goon** floo-hoh pohr lah vah-**hee**-nah)
9. Thick or thin?	¿Grueso o delgado?	(groo-**eh**-soh oh dehl-**gah**-doh)
10. What color?	¿Qué color?	(**keh** koh-**lohr**)

11. Yellow, white or gray?	¿Amarillo, blanco o gris?	(ahm-ahr-**ee**-yoh, **blahn**-koh, oh **grees**)
12. Do you use birth control?	¿Usa contraceptivos?	(oo-sah kohn-trah-sehp-**tee**-vohs)
13. Condoms?	¿Condones?	(kohn-**dohn**-ehs)
14. With nonoxynol 9?	¿Con nonoxynal nueve por ciento?	(kohn nohn-ohx-ee-**nahl** noo-**eh**-veh pohr see-**ehn**-toh)
15. Foam?	¿Crema o espuma?	(**kreh**-mah oh ehs-**poo**-mah)
16. Pills?	¿Pastillas o píldoras?	(pahs-**tee**-yahs oh **peel**-dohr-ahs)
17. Norplant?	¿Norplant?	(nohr-**plahnt**)
18. Diaphragm?	¿Diafragma?	(dee-ah-**frahg**-mah)
19. IUD?	¿Dispositivo intrauterino?	(dees-pohs-ee-**tee**-voh een-trah-oo-tehr-**een**-oh)

PAST MEDICAL HISTORY (PMH)

1. Do you have diabetes?	¿Tiene diabetes?	(tee-**ehn**-eh **dee**-ah-beh-tehs)
2. Do you have hypertension?	¿Tiene hipertensión?	(tee-**ehn**-eh ee-pehr-tehn-see-**ohn**)
3. Do you have asthma?	¿Tiene asma?	(tee-**ehn**-eh **ahs**-mah)
4. Do you have heart disease?	¿Tiene enfermedad del corazón?	(tee-**ehn**-eh ehn-fehr-meh-**dahd** dehl kohr-ah-**sohn**)
5. Rheumatic fever?	¿Fiebre reumática?	(fee-**eh**-breh reh-oo-**mah**-tee-kah)
6. Do you have a seizure disorder?	¿Tiene epilepsia o convulsiones?	(tee-**ehn**-eh eh-pee-lehp-**see**-ah oh kohn-vool-see-**ohn**-ehs)
7. Do you have any diseases?	¿Tiene algunas enfermedades?	(tee-**ehn**-eh ahl-**goo**-nahs ehn-fehr-meh-**dah**-dehs)

MEDICATION HISTORY

1. Are you taking any medications?	¿Toma algunas medicinas?	(**toh**-mah ahl-**goo**-nahs meh-dee-**see**-nahs)
2. What medicines?	¿Qué medicinas?	(**keh** meh-dee-**see**-nahs)
3. Prenatal vitamins?	¿Vitaminas prenatales?	(vee-tah-**mee**-nahs preh-nah-**tahl**-ehs)
4. Iron?	¿Hierro?	(hee-**ehr**-oh)

ALLERGIES

1. Do you have any allergies to medicines or food?	¿Tiene algunas alergias a las medicinas o comidas?	(tee-**ehn**-eh ahl-**goo**-nahs ahl-ehr-**hee**-ahs ah lahs meh-dee-**see**-nahs oh koh-**mee**-dahs)
2. What happens?	¿Qué ocurre?	(**keh** oh-**koo**-reh)

SOCIAL HISTORY

1. Are you working or going to school?	¿Trabaja o va a la escuela?	(trah-**bah**-hah oh vah lah ehs-koo-**eh**-lah)
2. Are you married or single?	¿Está casada o soltera?	(ehs-**tah** kah-**sah**-doh oh sohl-**tehr**-ah)
3. Is there anyone else that lives at home with you?	¿Alguna otra persona vive en su casa con usted?	(ahl-**goo**-nah oh-trah pehr-**sohn**-ah vee-veh ehn soo **kah**-sah kohn oos-**tehd**)
4. Have you drank any alcohol during this pregnancy?	¿Ha tomado alcohol durante este embarazo?	(ah toh-**mah**-doh ahl-koh-**ohl** doo-**rahn**-teh ehs-teh ehm-bahr-**ah**-soh)
5. How much?	¿Qué cantidad?	(**keh** kahn-tee-**dahd**)
6. A little or a lot?	¿Un poco o mucho?	(oon **poh**-koh oh **moo**-choh)
7. Do you smoke cigarettes?	¿Fuma cigarrillos?	(**foo**-mah see-gahr-**ee**-yohs)

8. How many cigarettes per day?	¿Cuántos cigarrillos al día?	(koo-**ahn**-tohs see-gahr-**ee**-yohs ahl **dee**-ah)
9. Do you use any drugs?	¿Usa algunas drogas?	(**oo**-sah ahl-**goo**-nahs **droh**-gahs)
10. Cocaine?	¿Cocaína?	(koh-kah-**een**-ah)
11. Heroin?	¿Heroína?	(ehr-oh-**een**-ah)

FAMILY HISTORY

1. Has anyone in your family had a baby with a birth defect?	¿Alguna persona en su familia ha tenido un bebé con defectos de nacimiento?	(ahl-**goo**-nah pehr-**sohn**-ah ehn soo fah-**meel**-ee-ah ah teh-**nee**-doh oon beh-**beh** kohn deh-**fehk**-tohs deh nah-see-mee-**ehn**-toh)
2. Mental retardation?	¿Retardado mental?	(reh-tahr-**dah**-doh mehn-**tahl**)
3. Does anyone in your family have diabetes?	¿Alguna persona en su familia tiene diabetes?	(ahl-**goo**-nah-pehr-**sohn**-ah ehn su fah-meel-ee-ah tee-**ehn**-eh **dee**-ah-bee-rehs)
4. Twins?	¿Gemelos?	(heh-**meh**-lohs)

REVIEW OF SYSTEMS

1. Do you have any pain or burning when you urinate?	¿Tiene dolor o ardor cuando orina?	(tee-**ehn**-eh doh-**lohr** oh ahr-**dohr** koo-**ahn**-doh oh-**ree**-nah)
2. Have you had a fever?	¿Ha tenido fiebre?	(ah teh-**nee**-doh fee-**eh**-breh)
3. Have you had a cold?	¿Ha tenido catarro?	(ah teh-**nee**-doh kah-**tah**-roh)
4. Do you have diarrhea?	¿Tiene diarrea?	(tee-**ehn**-eh dee-ahr-**ee**-ah)
5. Do you have a headache?	¿Tiene dolor de cabeza?	(tee-**ehn**-eh doh-**lohr** deh kah-**beh**-sah)

6. Have you had problems with your vision?	¿Ha tenido algún problema con su vista?	(ah teh-**nee**-doh ahl-**goon** proh-**bleh**-mah kohn soo **vees**-tah)
7. Do you have swelling of your feet?	¿Tiene hinchazón en los pies?	(tee-**ehn**-eh een-chah-**sohn** ehn los **pee**-ehs)
8. Your face or hands?	¿La cara o las manos?	(lah **kah**-rah oh lahs **mahn**-ohs)

ANTEPARTUM

1. How are you feeling?	¿Cómo se siente?	(**koh**-moh seh see-**ehn**-teh)
2. When is your due date?	¿Cuándo espera dar a luz?	(koo-**ahn**-doh ehs-**pehr**-ah dahr ah loos)
3. Are you having any contractions?	¿Tiene contracciones?	(tee-**ehn**-eh kohn-trak-see-**ohn**-ehs)
4. I need to measure the size of your abdomen (fundal height)	Necesito medir su abdomen	(neh-seh-**see**-toh meh-**deer** soo ahb-**doh**-mehn)
5. I need to listen to the heartbeat of the baby	Necesito escuchar los latidos del corazón del bebé	(neh-seh-**see**-toh ehs-koo-**chahr** lohs lah-**tee**-dohs dehl kohr-ah-**sohn** dehl beh-**beh**)
6. Do you want to listen?	¿Quiere escuchar?	(kee-**ehr**-eh ehs-koo-**chahr**)
7. You need a blood test	Necesita una prueba de sangre	(neh-seh-**see**-tah oo-nah proo-**eh**-bah deh **sahn**-gre)
8. You need a urine test	Necesita una prueba de orina	(neh-seh-**see**-tah oo-nah proo-**eh**-bah deh ohr-**ee**-nah)
9. You need an U/S	Necesita un ultrasonido	(neh-seh-**see**-tah oon ool-trah-soh-**nee**-doh)
10. You need a test to check the baby's heartbeat (NST)	Necesita una prueba para chequear los latidos del corazón del bebé	(neh-seh-**see**-tah oo-nah proo-**eh**-bah pah-rah cheh-keh-**ahr** lohs lah-**tee**-dohs dehl kohr-ah-**sohn** dehl beh-**beh**)

11. Return to the clinic in two weeks	Regrese a la clínica en dos semanas	(reh-**greh**-seh ah lah **klee**-nee-kah ehn dohs seh-**mahn**-ahs)

LABOR AND DELIVERY

1. See earlier chapters for H & P format

2. Do you want to go to the bathroom?	¿Quiere ir al baño?	(kee-**ehr**-eh eer ahl **bah**-nyoh)
3. Do you want the bedpan?	¿Quiere usar la basinilla?	(kee-**ehr**-eh oo-**sahr** lah bah-seen-**ee**-yah)
4. Do you want to get up and walk now?	¿Quiere levantarse y caminar ahora?	(kee-**ehr**-eh leh-vahn-**tahr**-seh ee kah-mee-**nahr** ah-**ohr**-ah)
5. Enema	Enema	(ehn-**eh**-mah)

CERVICAL EXAM

1. Cervix	La cerviz o el cuello de la matriz	(lah sehr-**vees** oh ehl koo-**eh**-yoh deh lah mah-**trees**)
2. Open your legs more	Abra sus piernas más	(**ah**-brah soos pee-**ehr**-nahs **mahs**)
3. Centimeters	Centímetros	(sehn-**tee**-meh-trohs)
4. You are 3 centimeters dilated	Usted tiene tres centímetros de dilatación	(oos-**tehd** tee-**ehn**-eh trehs sehn-**tee**-meh-trohs deh dee-lah-tah-see-**ohn**)
5. Open	Abierto	(ah-bee-**ehr**-toh)
6. Closed	Cerrado	(seh-**rah**-doh)
7. High	Alto	(**ahl**-toh)
8. Low	Bajo	(**bah**-hoh)
9. Thick	Grueso	(groo-**eh**-soh)
10. Thin	Delgado	(dehl-**gah**-doh)

TECHNICAL TERMS

1. Bag of Water (Bow)	La bolsa de agua	(lah **bohl**-sah deh ah-**goo**-ah)
2. FHTs	Los latidos del corazón del bebé	(lohs lah-**tee**-dohs dehl koh-rah-**sohn** dehl beh-**beh**)
3. Meconium	El bebé defecó antes de nacer	(ehl beh-**beh** deh-feh-**koh** ahn-tehs deh nah-**sehr**)
4. IUPC	Es una sonda para medir las contracciones	(ehs oo-nah **sohn**-dah pah-rah meh-**deer** las kohn-trak-see-**ohn**-ehs)
5. FSE	Es un alambrito para medir los latidos	(ehs oon ah-lahm-**bree**-toh pah-rah meh-**deer** lohs lah-**tee**-dohs)
6. IVF	Suero	(soo-**ehr**-oh)
7. Pitocin	Medicina a través por del suero para aumentar las contracciones	(meh-dee-**see**-nah ah trah-vehs pohr dehl soo-**ehr**-oh pah-rah ah-oo-mehn-**tahr** lahs kohn-trak-see-**ohn**-ehs)

PUSHING INSTRUCTIONS

1. Relax	Relájese	(reh-**lah**-heh-seh)
2. Push	Puje	(**poo**-heh)
3. Hold your breath and push	Aguante su respiración y puje	(ah-goo-**ahn**-teh soo rehs-peer-ah-see-**ohn** ee **poo**-heh)
4. Don't let the air out when you push	No suelte el aire cuando puje	(noh soo-**ehl**-teh ehl ah-**ee**-reh koo-**ahn**-doh **poo**-heh)
5. Push harder	Más fuerte	(**mahs** foo-**ehr**-teh)
6. Push again	Puje otra vez	(**poo**-heh **oh**-trah vehs)
7. More	Más	(**mahs**)
8. Good job	Muy bien	(moo-ee bee-**ehn**)

9. Rest between contractions	Descanse entre contracciones	(dehs-cah-**on**-seh ehn-treh kohn-trahk-see-**ohn**-ehs)
10. Push as if you were going to have a bowel movement	Puje como si fuera a defecar	(**poo**-heh **koh**-moh see foo-**ehr**-ah ah deh-feh-**kahr**)
11. Lift your hips	Levante sus caderas	(ye-**vahn**-teh soos kah-**deh**-rahs)
12. I need to check for dilatation	Necesito chequear la dilatación	(neh-seh-**see**-toh cheh-keh-**ahr** lah dee-lah-tah-see-**ohn**)
13. It is time to move to the delivery room	Es tiempo de llevarla a la sala de partos	(ehs tee-**ehm**-poh deh yeh-**vahr**-lah ah lah **sah**-lah deh **pahr**-tohs)
14. Put your chin to your chest	Ponga su barbilla en su pecho	(**pohn**-gah soo bahr-**bee**-yah ehn soo **peh**-choh)

DELIVERY ROOM

1. Don't push	No puje	(noh **poo**-heh)
2. Breathe	Respire	(reh-**spee**-reh)
3. Put your legs here	Ponga las piernas aquí	(**pohn**-gah lahs pee-**ehr**-nahs ah-**kee**)
4. Move down more	Muévase más de abajo	(moo-**eh**-vah-seh **mahs** deh ah-**bah**-hoh)
5. Push	Puje	(**poo**-heh)
6. The head is coming	Aquí viene la cabeza	(ah-**kee** vee-**ehn**-eh lah kah-**beh**-sah)
7. It's a boy!	¡Es un niño!	(ehs oon **nee**-nyoh)
8. It's a girl!	¡Es una niña!	(ehs oon-ah **nee**-nyah)
9. Pounds (lbs)	Libras	(**lee**-brahs)
10. Ounces (oz)	Onzas	(**ohn**-sahs)

11. Congratulations!	¡Felicitaciones!	(feh-lee-see-tah-see-**ohn**-ehs)
12. Laceration	Una laceración	(oon-ah lah-seh-rah-see-**ohn**)
13. Episiotomy	Una episiotomía	(oon-ah eh-pees-see-oh-toh-**mee**-ah)
14. Incision	Una incisión	(oon-ah een-see-see-**ohn**)
15. You will feel a little stick	Sentirá un pinchazo	(sehn-teer-**ah** oon peen-**chah**-so)
16. Placenta	Placenta	(plah-**sehn**-tah)
17. This is to clean you	Esto es para limpiarle	(ehs-toh ehs pah-rah leem-pee-**ahr**-leh)
18. A little cold	Un poco frío	(oon **poh**-koh **free**-oh)
19. Blanket	La manta	(lah **mahn**-tah)
20. Incubator	Incubadora	(een-koo-bah-**dohr**-ah)
21. Pediatrician	Pediatra	(peh-dee-**ah**-trah)
22. Recovery room	La sala de recuperación	(lah **sah**-lah deh reh-koo-pehr-ah-see-**ohn**)
23. Nursery	La enfermería	(lah ehn-fehr-meh-**ree**-ah)
24. Sanitary napkin	Toalla sanitaria	(toh-**ah**-yah sahn-ee-tahr-**ee**-ah)

FETAL DISTRESS

1. Turn on your side	Póngase de lado	(**pohn**-gah-seh deh **lah**-doh)
2. Left	Izquierda	(ees-kee-**ehr**-dah)
3. Right	Derecha	(deh-**reh**-chah)
4. Oxygen	Oxígeno	(ohx-**ee**-heh-noh)
5. It is better for the baby	Es mejor para el bebé	(ehs meh-**hor** pah-rah ehl beh-**beh**)
6. Your baby is very sick	Su bebé está muy enfermo	(soo beh-**beh** ehs-**tah** moo-ee ehn-**fehr**-moh)

CESAREAN SECTION

1. Cesarean section	Operación cesárea	(oh-pehr-ah-see-**ohn** seh-**sahr**-ee-ah)
2. The risks are bleeding, infection	Los riesgos son hemorragia, infección	(lohs ree-**ehs**-gohs sohn ehm-ohr-ah-**hee**-ah een-fehk-see-**ohn**)
3. And injuries to the bladder and bowel	y daños en la vejiga y el intestino	(ee **dahn**-ohs ehn lah veh-**hee**-gah ee ehl een-tehs-**teen**-oh)
4. Also, fetus reaction to anesthesia	También, reacción del feto a la anestesia	(tahm-bee-**ehn**, reh-ahk-see-**ohn** dehl **feh**-toh ah lah ahn-ehs-tehs-**ee**-ah)
5. If there is severe bleeding	Si hay hemorragia severa	(see eye ehm-ohr-ah-**hee**-ah seh-**vehr** ah)
6. You may need to have your uterus removed	Es posible que tengamos que remover el utero	(ehs pos-**see**-bleh keh tehn-**gah**-mohs keh reh-moh-**vehr** ehl oo-**tehr**-oh)
7. You may need to have a blood transfusion	Es posible que necesitará una transfusión de sangre	(ehs poh-**see**-bleh keh neh-seh-see-tah-**rah** oon-ah trahns-foo-see-**ohn** deh **sahn**-greh)
8. The blood is screened for HIV and hepatitis	Toda la sangre esta analizada para SIDA y hepatitis	(**toh**-dah lah **sahn**-gre ehs-tah ahn-ah-lee-**sah**-dah pah-rah **see**-dah ee eh-pah-**tee**-tees)
9. Do you understand?	¿Entiende?	(ehn-tee-**ehn**-deh)

POSTOP CESAREAN SECTION

1. Foley catheter	La sonda vesical o la sonda de la orina	(lah **sohn**-dah veh-see-**kahl** oh lah **sohn**-dah deh lah oh-**ree**-nah)
2. We will take out the catheter	Quitaremos la sonda	(kee-tahr-**ehm**-ohs lah **sohn**-dah)
3. Incentive spirometry	Espirómetro	(ehs-peer-**oh**-meh-troh)

4. Get out of bed and try to walk	Levántese de la cama y trate de caminar	(leh-**vahn**-teh-seh deh lah **kah**-mah ee **trah**-teh deh kah-mee-**nahr**)
5. No oral food	No tome nada por la boca	(noh **toh**-meh **nah**-dah pohr lah **boh**-kah)
6. Clear liquids	Líquidos claros	(**lee**-kee-dohs **klah**-rohs)
7. Soft food diet	Dieta blanda	(dee-**eh**-tah **blahn**-dah)
8. Remove staples	Quitar grapas	(kee-**tahr grah**-pahs)
9. Have you moved your bowels?	¿Ha evacuado el intestino?	(ah eh-vah-koo-**ah**-doh ehl een-tehs-**tee**-noh)
10. Wound separation with drainage?	¿Separación de la herida con drenaje?	(seh-pahr-ah-see-**ohn** deh lah ehr-**ee**-dah kohn drehn-**ah**-heh)

POSTPARTUM FOLLOW UP AND DISCHARGE

1. How are you feeling?	¿Cómo se siente?	(**koh**-moh seh see-**ehn**-teh)
2. Any problems?	¿Algún problema?	(ahl-**goon** proh-**bleh**-mahs)
3. Are you going to breastfeed or bottlefeed?	¿Le va a dar pecho o botella?	(leh vah ah dahr **peh**-choh oh boh-**teh**-yah)
4. Is the bleeding slowing down?	¿Sangra menos por la vagina?	(**sahn**-grah **meh**-nos pohr-lah vah-**hee**-nah)
5. How many pads?	¿Cuántas toallas sanitarias?	(koo-**ahn**-tahs toh-**ah**-yahs sahn-ee-tahr-**ee**-ahs)
6. Do you have pain in your breasts?	¿Tiene dolor en los pechos?	(tee-**ehn**-eh doh-**lohr** ehn lohs **peh**-chohs)
7. A tight bra and an ice pack will help relieve this	Un brassiere bastante apretado y una bolsa de hielo ayudan	(oon brah-see-**ehr**-eh bahs-**tahn**-teh ah-preh-**tah**-doh ee oon-ah **bohl**-sah deh ee-**eh**-loh eye-yoo-**dahn**)

8. Rubella vaccine	La vacuna de Rubéola	(lah vah-**koon**-ah deh roo-**beh**-oh-lah)
9. Nothing in the vagina for six weeks	Nada por la vagina por seis semanas	(**nah**-dah pohr lah vah-**hee**-nah pohr seh-**ees** seh-**mah**-nahs)
10. No sex, douche, or tampons	Nada de sexo, ducha, o tampones	(**nah**-dah deh **sehx**-oh **doo**-chah oh tahm-**pohn**-ehs)
11. It is important to use contraception	Es importante que use contraceptivos	(ehs eem-pohr-**tahn** teh keh **oo**-sah kohn-trah-sehp-**tee**-vos)
12. When you start having sexual intercourse again	Cuando comienze relaciones sexuales de nuevo	(koo-**ahn**-doh koh-mee-**ehn**-seh reh-lah-see-**ohn**-ehs sehx-oo-**ahl**-ehs deh noo-**eh**-voh)
13. Be careful when you drive	Tenga cuidado cuando maneje el coche	(**tehn**-gah koo-ee-**dah**-doh koo-**ahn**-doh mahn-**eh**-heh ehl **koh**-cheh)
14. You will be discharged today	Le vamos a dar de alta hoy	(leh **vah**-mohs ah dahr deh **ahl**-tah oy)
15. You will be discharged tomorrow	Le vamos a dar de alta mañana	(leh **vah**-mos ah dahr deh ahl-tah mah-**nyah**-nah)
16. Come to the clinic in six weeks	Vuelva a la clínica en seis semanas	(voo-**ehl**-vah ah lah **kleen**-ee-kah ehn seh-**ees** seh-**mahn**-ahs)

CIRCUMCISION

1. Do you want the baby to be circumcised?	¿Quiere circuncidar al bebé?	(kee-**ehr**-eh seer-koon-see-**dahr** ahl beh-**beh**)
2. There are no medical reasons to circumcise or not circumcise	No hay razón médica para circuncidar o no circuncidar	(noh eye rah-**sohn meh**-dee-kah pah-rah seer-koon-see-**dahr** oh noh seer-koon-see-**dahr**)

3. His penis will look red and swollen for a few days	El pene se va a ver rojo e hinchado por unos días	(ehl **peh**-neh seh vah ah vehr **roh**-hoh eh een-**chah**-doh pohr oon-ohs **dee**-ahs)
4. If it bleeds, hold pressure with a gauze with vaseline	Si sangra, aguante la presión con gasa y vaselina	(see **sahn**-grah, ah-goo-**ahn**-teh lah preh-see-**ohn** kohn **gah**-sah ee vah-seh-**lee**-nah)
5. Call the pediatrician if it looks infected	Llame al pediatra si se ve infectado	(**yah**-meh ahl peh-dee-**ah**-trah see seh veh een-fehk-**tah**-doh)

TUBAL LIGATION

1. Are you sure you want a tubal ligation?	¿Está segura que quiere una ligadura de las trompas?	(eh-**stah** seh-**goo**-rah keh kee-**ehr**-eh oon-ah lee-gah-**doo**-rah deh lahs **trohm**-pahs)
2. It is permanent	Es permanente	(ehs pehr-mahn-**ehn**-teh)
3. 1 out of 250 women become pregnant after a tubal ligation	En una de cada doscientas cincuenta mujeres la operación falla y el embarazo ocurre	(ehn oon-ah deh **cah**-dah dohs-see-**ehn**-tahs seen-koo-**ehn**-tah moo-**hehr**-ehs lah oh-pehr-ah-see-**ohn** fah-yah ee ehl ehm-bahr-**ah**-soh oh-**koo**-reh)
4. It is very rare but an ectopic pregnancy could occur	Es muy raro pero un embarazo ectópico puede ocurrir	(ehs moo-ee **rahr**-oh **pehr**-oh oon ehm-bah-**rah**-soh ehk-**toh**-pee-koh poo-**eh**-deh oh-koo-**reer**)

AMNIOCENTESIS

Indications

1. The purpose of this test	El propósito de esta prueba	(ehl proh-**pohs**-ee-toh deh ehs-tah proo-**eh**-bah)

2. Is to look for chromosome (CS) abnormalities	Es para buscar anormalidades de cromosomas	(ehs pah-rah boos-**kahr** ah-nohr-mah-lee-**dah**-des deh kroh-moh-**soh**-mahs)
3. Children of women more than 35 years old	Hijos de mujeres mayores de treinta y cinco años	(**ee**-hohs deh moo-**hehr**-ehs meye-**ohr**-ehs deh **trehn**-tah ee **seen**-koh **ah**-nyohs)
4. Have a higher risk of having Down syndrome	Tienen mayor risego del síndrome de Down	(tee-**ehn**-ehn meye-**ohr** ree-**ehs**-goh dehl **seen**-droh-meh deh **dohwn**)
5. Children of women with decreased levels of alpha-feto protein	Hijos de mujeres con niveles disminuido de alfa-fetoproteína	(**ee**-hohs deh moo-**hehr**-ehs kohn nee-**veh**-lehs dees-meen-oo-ee-doh deh **ahl**-fah-feh-toh-proh-teh-**ee**-nah)
6. Have a higher risk of Down's Syndrome	Tienen mayor riesgo del síndrome de Down	(tee-**ehn**-ehn meye-**ohr** ree-**ehs**-goh dehl seen-**dro**-meh dohwn)
7. U/S is able to detect the majority of congenital abnormalities	El ultrasonido puede detectar la mayoría de las anormalidades congenitales	(ehl ool-trah-soh-**nee**-doh poo-**eh**-deh deh-tehk-**tahr** lah meye-ohr-**ee**-ah deh lahs ah-nohr-mahl-ee-**dah**-dehs kohn-heh-**nee**-tahl-ehs)
8. However, there are some abnormalities which are not able to be detected with U/S	Sin embargo, existen algunas anormalidades que no pueden ser detectadas	(seen ehm-**bahr**-goh, ehx-**ees**-tehn ahl-**goo**-nahs ah-nohr-mah-ee-**dah**-dehs keh noh poo-**eh**-dehn sehr deh-tehk-**tah**-dahs)
9. On the U/S your baby has choroid plexus cyst	En el ultrasonido su bebé tiene un quiste del plexo choroide del cerebro	(ehn ehl ool-trah-soh-**nee**-doh soo beh-**beh** tee-**ehn**-eh oon **kees**-teh dehl **plehx**-oh koh-roh-**ee**-deh del sehr-**eh**-broh)
10. This is sometimes associated with CS abnormalities	Estos es a veces asociado con anormalidades de cromosomas	(eh-stoh ehs ah veh-sehs ah-soh-see-**ah**-doh kohn ah-nohr-mahl-ee-**dah**-dehs deh kroh-moh-**soh**-mahs)

Explanation of Procedure and Risks

1. With this procedure about 1/200 women have the risk of losing their baby	Con este procedimiento una de cada dos cientos mujeres tiene el riesgo de perder su bebé	(kohn ehs-teh proh-seh-dee-mee-**ehn**-toh oon-ah deh **kah**-dah dohs-see-**ehn**-tohs moo-**jehr**-ehs tee-**ehn**-eh ehl ree-**ehs**-koh deh pehr-**dehr** soo beh-**beh**)
2. Amniotic fluid is the liquid around the baby	El líquido amniótico es el líquido alrededor del bebé	(ehl **lee**-kee-doh ahm-nee-**oh**-tee-koh ehs ehl **lee**-kee-doh ahl-reh-deh-**dohr** dehl beh-**beh**)
3. I will use U/S to guide the needle into the fluid	Usaré el ultrasonido para guiar la aguja dentro del líquido	(oo-sahr-**eh** ehl ool-trah-sohn-**ee**-doh pah-rah gee-**ahr** lah ah-**goo**-hah **dehn**-troh dehl **lee**-kee-doh)
4. And to avoid the baby	Y para evitar el bebé	(ee pah-rah eh-vee-**tahr** ehl beh-**beh**)
5. A small amout of amniotic fluid will be removed	Un cantidad pequeña de líquido amniótico removerá	(oon kahn-tee-**dahd** peh-**keh**-nyah deh **lee**-kee-doh ahm-nee-**oh**-tee-koh reh-moh-vehr-**ah**)
6. And then sent to the laboratory for analysis	Y entonces lleva al laboratorio para análisis	(ee ehn-**tohn**-sehs **yeh**-vah ah lah lah-bohr-oh-**tohr**-ee-oh pah-rah ahn-**ah**-lee-sees)
7. The procedure usually takes 10 minutes or less	Este procedimiento usualmente lleva diez minutos o menos	(ehs-teh proh-seh-dee-mee-**ehn**-toh oos-oo-ahl-**mehn**-teh yeh-vah dee-**ehs** mee-**noo**-tohs oh **meh**-nohs)
8. I will give you local anesthesia to minimize the pain	Le daré anestesia local para disminuir su dolor	(leh dah-**reh** ahn-eh-stehs-**ee**-ah loh-kahl pah-rah dees-meen-oo-**eer** soo doh-**lohr**)

9. It will still hurt a little bit	No puedo prevenir el dolor completamente	(noh poo-**eh**-doh preh-veh-**neer** ehl doh-**lohr** kohm-pleh-tah-**mehn**-teh)
10. I can't put local anesthesia into the uterus because of the baby	No puedo ponerle anestesia local en el útero para el beneficio del bebé	(noh poo-**eh**-doh poh-**nehr**-leh ahn-ehs-tehs-**ee**-ah loh-**kahl** ehn ehl **oo**-teh-roh pah-rah ehl beh-neh-fee-**see**-oh dehl beh-**beh**)
11. You will feel a slight cramp/pinch	Sentirá un ligero calambre o pinchazo	(sehn-tee-**rah** oon lee-**geh**-roh kah-**lahm**-breh oh peen-**cha**-soh)
12. When the needle goes into the uterus	Cuando la aguja entre en su útero	(koo-**ahn**-doh lah ah-**goo**-hah ehn-treh ehn soo **oo**-teh-roh)
13. Please do not move when the needle is inside	Por favor no se mueva cuando la aguja esté adentro	(pohr fah-**vohr** nos seh moo-**eh**-vah koo-**ahn**-doh lah ah-**goo**-ha ehs-**teh** ah-**dehn**-troh)

Postprocedure Instructions

1. You should not have more pain than you are having now	No debe tener mas dolor del que tiene ahora	(noh deh-beh teh-**nehr** mahs doh-**lohr** dehl keh tee-**ehn**-eh ah-**ohr**-ah)
2. If you start to have more pain, you should call your doctor	Si tiene mas dolor debe llamar a su doctor	(see tee-**ehn**-eh mahs doh-**lohr** deh-beh **yah**-mahr ah soo dohk-**tohr**)
3. You should avoid strenuous activity for 3 days	Debe evitar actividades fuertes por tres días	(deh-beh eh-vee-**tahr** ahk-tee-vee-**dah**-dehs foo-**ehr**-tehs pohr trehs **dee**-ahs)
4. The results will be available in 2 to 3 weeks	Los resultados estarán listos en dos o tres semanas	(lohs reh-sool-**tah**-dohs ehs-tahr-**ahn** lees-tohs ehn dohs oh trehs seh-**mah**-nahs)

2. PEDIATRICS

CHAPTER OUTLINE

Age	Shortness of Breath	Rash
Fever	Vomiting	Nutrition
Cough	Ear Pain	Immunizations
Nasal Discharge	Diarrhea	

AGE

1. How old is the child (years)?	¿Cuántos años tiene el niño?	(koo-**ahn**-tohs **ah**-nyohs tee-**ehn**-eh ehl **nee**-nyoh)
2. How old is the baby (mos.)?	¿Cuántos meses tiene el bebé?	(koo-**ahn**-tohs **meh**-sehs tee-**eh**-neh ehl beh-**beh**)
3. How old is the baby (wks.)?	¿Cuántas semanas tiene el bebé?	(koo-**ahn**-tas seh-**mahn**-ahs tee-**eh**-neh ehl beh-**beh**)

FEVER

1. How many days have you had a fever?	¿Cuántos días ha tenido fiebre?	(koo-**ahn**-tohs **dee**-ahs hah teh-**nee**-doh fee-**eh**-breh)
2. What was the temperature?	¿Cuál fue la temperatura?	(koo-**ahl** foo-eh lah tehm-pehr-ah-**too**-rah)
3. Do you have a thermometer?	¿Tiene un termómetro?	(tee-**ehn**-eh oon tehr-**moh**-meh-troh)
4. Did you just touch his forehead?	¿Solamente le tocó la frente?	(soh-lah-**mehn**-teh leh toh-**koh** lah-**frehn**-teh)

5. Was it very hot?	¿Estaba muy caliente?	(ehs-**tah**-bah moo-ee kah-lee-**ehn**-teh)
6. Was it only a little hot?	¿Estaba solamente un poco caliente?	(ehs-**tah**-bah soh-lah-**mehn**-teh oon **poh**-koh kah-lee-**ehn**-teh)
7. Does anyone else in the family have a fever?	¿Algunas otras personas en su familia tienen fiebre?	(ahl-**goon**-ahs oh-trahs pehr-**soh**-nahs ehn soo fah-mee-**lee**-ah tee-**ehn**-ehn fee-**eh**-breh)
8. Does anyone else have the same symptoms?	¿Algunas otras personas tienen los mismos síntomas?	(ahl-**goon**-ahs oh-trahs pehr-**soh**-nahs tee-**ehn**-ehn lohs **mees**-mohs **seen**-toh-mahs)

COUGH

1. Do you have a cough?	¿Tiene tos?	(tee-**eh**-neh tohs)
2. How many days have you had a cough?	¿Cuántos días ha tenido tos?	(koo-**ahn**-tohs **dee**-ahs ah teh-**nee**-doh tohs)
3. How often do you cough?	¿Con qué frequencia?	(kohn **keh** freh-koo-ehn-**see**-ah)
4. Is there a lot of mucus or phlegm?	¿Con mucho moco o flema?	(kohn moo-cho **moh**-choh oh **fleh**-mah)
5. What color?	¿Qué color?	(**keh** koh-**lohr**)
6. Yellow, gray, or green?	¿Amarillo, gris o verde?	(ahm-ahr-**ee**-yoh, **grees**, oh **vehr**-deh)

NASAL DISCHARGE

1. Do you have nasal discharge?	¿Tiene flujo por la nariz?	(tee-**eh**-neh **floo**-hoh pohr lah nah-**rees**)
2. A lot or a little?	¿Mucho o poco?	(**moo**-choh oh **poh**-koh)

SHORTNESS OF BREATH

1. Do you have difficulty breathing?	¿Tiene dificultad al respirar?	(tee-**eh**-neh dee-fee-kool-**tahd** ahl rehs-peer-**ahr**)
2. Do you have asthma?	¿Tiene asma?	(tee-**eh**-neh **ahs**-mah)
3. Do you have wheezing?	¿Tiene silbido?	(tee-**eh**-neh seel-**bee**-doh)

VOMITING

1. How many days have you been vomiting?	¿Cuántos días ha tenido vomitos?	(koo-**ahn**-tohs **dee**-ahs ah teh-**nee**-doh voh-**mee**-tohs)
2. How many times today?	¿Cuántas veces hoy?	(koo-**ahn**-tas **veh**-sees oy)
3. How many times yesterday?	¿Cuántas veces ayer?	(koo-**ahn**-tas **veh**-sees eye-**ehr**)
4. When do you vomit?	¿Cuándo vomita?	(koo-**ahn**-doh voh-**mee**-tah)
5. After meals?	¿Después de la comida?	(dehs-poo-**ehs** deh lah koh-**mee**-dah)
6. After coughing?	¿Después de la tos?	(dehs-poo-**ehs** deh lah tohs)
7. In the morning?	¿En la mañana?	(ehn lah mahn-**nyah**-nah)
8. What color is it?	¿De qué color es el vómito?	(deh **keh** koh-**lohr** ehs ehl **voh**-mee-toh)
9. Green, brown or red?	¿Verde, marrón o rojo?	(**vehr**-deh mah-**rohn** oh **roh**-hoh)
10. Did it contain blood?	¿Con sangre?	(kohn **sahn**-greh)

EAR PAIN

1. Do you have pain in your ears?	¿Tiene dolor en los oídos?	(tee-**eh**-neh doh-**lohr** ehn lohs oh-**ee**-dohs)
2. Right, left, or both?	¿El derecho, izquierdo, o ambos?	(lah deh-**reh**-choh ees-kee-**ehr**-doh o **ahm**-bohs)

3. Which is worse?	¿Cuál está peor?	(koo-**ahl** ehs-**tah** peh-**ohr**)
4. How many days have you had ear pain?	¿Cuántos días ha tenido dolor en el oído?	(koo-**ahn**-tohs **dee**-ahs ah teh-**nee**-doh doh-**lohr** ehn ehl oh-**ee**-doh)
5. Do you have difficulty hearing?	¿Tiene dificultad al oir?	(tee-**eh**-neh dee-fee-kool-**tahd** ahl oh-**eer**)
6. Do you hear well?	¿Oye bien?	(oy-eh bee-**ehn**)

DIARRHEA

1. Do you have diarrhea?	¿Tiene diarrea?	(tee-**eh**-neh **dee**-ahr-reh-ah)
2. How many stools today?	¿Cuántos excrementos hoy?	(koo-**ahn**-tohs ehx-kreh-**mehn**-tohs oy)
3. How many stools yesterday?	¿Cuántos excrementos ayer?	(koo-**ahn**-tohs ehx-kreh-**mehn**-tohs eye-**yehr**)
4. What is the normal number for this child?	¿Cuál es el número normal para este niño?	(koo-**ahl** ehs ehl **noo**-merh-roh nohr-**mahl** pah-rah ehs-teh **nee**-nyoh)
5. What color are the stools?	¿De qué color es el excremento?	(deh **keh** koh-**lohr** ehs ehl ehx-kreh-**mehn**-toh)
6. Do the stools contain blood?	¿Con sangre?	(kohn **sahn**-gre)
7. Do the stools contain a lot of mucus?	¿Con muchos mocos?	(kohn **moo**-chohs **moh**-kohs)

RASH

1. Do you have a rash?	¿Tiene una erupción?	(tee-**eh**-neh oo-nah eh-roop-see-**ohn**)
2. Where is the rash?	¿Dónde está la erupción?	(**dohn**-deh ehs-**tah** lah eh-roop-see-**ohn**)

3. Does it itch?	¿Tiene picazón?	(tee-**eh**-neh pee-kah-**sohn**)
4. Do not scratch it	No se rasque	(noh seh **rahs**-keh)

NUTRITION

1. Does the baby eat well?	¿Come bien el bebé?	(**koh**-meh bee-**ehn** ehl beh-**beh**)
2. From the breast or from the bottle?	¿Del pecho o de la botella?	(dehl **peh**-cho oh deh lah boh-**tey**-yah)
3. How many times per day?	¿Cuántas veces al día?	(koo-**ahn**-tahs veh-sehs ahl **dee**-ah)
4. Breakfast	Desayuno	(dehs-eye-**oo**-noh)
5. Lunch	Almuerzo	(ahl-moo-**ehr**-soh)
6. Dinner	Cena	(**seh**-nah)
7. How many ounces with each meal?	¿Cuántas onzas por cada comida?	(koo-**ahn**-tahs ohn-sahs pohr **kah**-dah koh-**mee**-dah)
8. Banana	Banana	(bah-**nah**-nah)
9. Rice	Arroz	(**ah**-rohs)
10. Apple	Manzana	(mahn-**sahn**-ah)
11. Toast	Pan tostado	(pahn toh-**stah**-doh)

IMMUNIZATIONS

1. Does the child have his/her vaccinations?	¿Tiene las vacunas?	(tee-**eh**-neh lahs vah-**koo**-nahs)
2. Do you have the form for the vaccinations?	¿Tiene la forma para las vacunas?	(tee-**eh**-neh lah **fohr**-mah pah-rah lahs vah-**koo**-nahs)
3. Diphtheria	Difteria	(deef-teh-**ree**-ah)
4. Pertussis	Tosferina	(tohs-feh-**ree**-nah)
5. Tetanus	Tétano	(**teh**-tahn-oh)

6. Polio, taken orally	Polio, por la boca	(poh-**lee**-oh, pohr lah **boh**-kah)
7. Measles	Sarampión	(sah-rahm-pee-**ohn**)
8. Mumps	Papera	(pah-**peh**-rah)
9. Rubella	Rubeóla	(roo-beh-**oh**-lah)
10. Skin test for tuberculosis	La prueba cutánea de tuberculina	(lah proo-**eh**-bah koo-**tahn**-eh-ah deh too-behr-koo-**lee**-nah)

3. OPHTHALMOLOGY

CHAPTER OUTLINE

ANATOMY

1. Choroid	Coroides	(koh-**roy**-dehs)
2. Conjunctiva	Conjuntiva	(kohn-joon-**tee**-vah)
3. Cornea	Córnea	(**kohr**-neh-ah)
4. Eye	Ojo	(**oh**-hoh)
5. Eyebrow	Ceja	(**seh**-hah)
6. Eyelashes	Pestañas	(pehs-**tah**-nahs)
7. Eyelids	Párpados	(**pahr**-pah-dohs)
8. Eye muscles	Músculos del ojo	(**moos**-koo-lohs dehl **oh**-hoh)

9. Iris	Iris	(**ee**-rees)
10. Lens	Cristalino	(krees-tah-**lee**-noh)
11. Orbit	Orbita	(ohr-**bee**-tah)
12. Pupil	Pupila	(poo-**pee**-lah)
13. Retina	Retina	(reh-**teen**-ah)
14. Sclera	Esclerótica	(ehs-klehr-**oh**-tee-kah)
15. Tear ducts	Orificio lagrimal	(oh-ree-fee-**see**-oh lah-gree-**mahl**)
16. Tears	Lágrimas	(**lah**-gree-mahs)
17. Uvea	Uvea	(oo-**veh**-ah)
18. Vitreous	Vítreo	(**vee**-treh-oh)

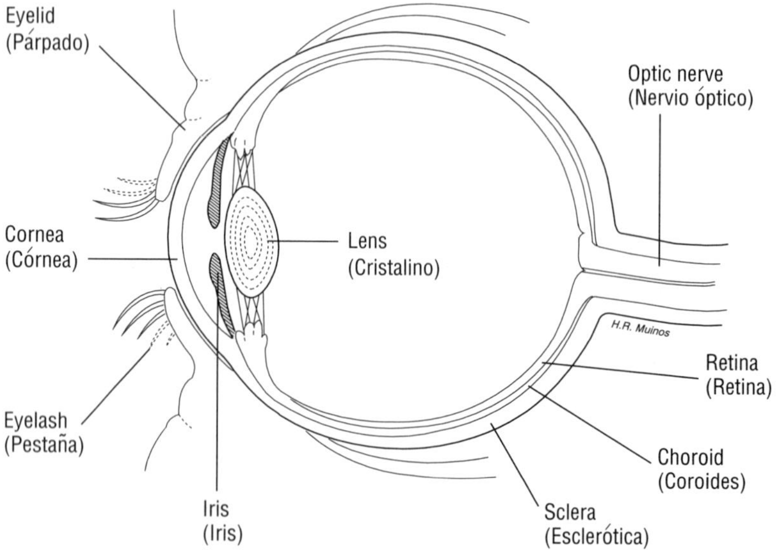

Figure 3. The eye (side view).

COMMON PROBLEMS

1. Red eye	Ojo rojo	(**oh**-hoh **roh**-hoh)
2. Conjunctivitis	Conjuntivitis	(kohn-joon-tee-**vee**-tees)
3. High pressure in the eye	La presión alta en el ojo	(lah preh-see-**ohn** ahl-tah ehn ehl **oh**-hoh)
4. Glaucoma	Glaucoma	(glah-oo-**koh**-mah)
5. Headache	Dolor de cabeza	(doh-**lohr** deh kah-**beh**-sah)
6. Detached retina	Desgarro de la retina	(dehs-**gah**-roh deh lah reh-**teen**-ah)
7. Corneal abrasion	Abrasión de la córnea	(ah-brah-see-**ohn** deh lah **kohr**-neh-ah)
8. Seeing double	Viendo doble	(vee-**ehn**-doh **doh**-bleh)

COMMON QUESTIONS

1. Does your eye hurt?	¿Le duele su ojo?	(leh doo-**eh**-leh soo **oh**-hoh)
2. Is your eye red?	¿Está su ojo rojo?	(ehs-**tah** soo **oh**-hoh **roh**-hoh)
3. Is there discharge from your eye?	¿Secreta su ojo alguna substancia anormal?	(Seh-**kreh**-tah soo **oh**-hoh ahl-**goon**-ah soob-stahn-**see**-ah ah-nohr-**mahl**)
4. What color is the discharge?	¿De qué color es la secreción?	(deh **keh** koh-**lohr** ehs ehl seh-kreh-see-**ohn**)
5. Are your eyelids stuck together in the morning?	¿Están sus parpados pegados por la mañana?	(ehs-**tahn** soos pahr-**pah**-dohs peh-**gah**-dohs pohr lah mah-**nyah**-nah)
6. Do you feel like there is something in your eye?	¿Siente como si tuviera algo en su ojo?	(see-**ehn**-teh **koh**-moh see too-vee-**ehr**-ah ahl-goh ehn soo **oh**-hoh)
7. Did something scratch your eye?	¿Algo rasguñó su ojo?	(ahl-goh rahs-goo-**nyoh** soo **oh**-hoh)

8. Did you get any chemicals in your eye?	¿Le entró algun elemento químico en su ojo?	(leh ehn-**troh** ahl-**goon** ehl-eh-**mehn**-toh **kee**-mee-koh ehn soo **oh**-hoh)
9. Are you seeing flashes of lights?	¿Ve flashes de luces?	(veh **flah**-shehs deh **loo**-sehs)
10. Do you have allergies?	¿Tiene alergias?	(tee-**ehn**-eh ah-lehr-**hee**-ahs)
11. Do you have any medical problems?	¿Tiene problemas?	(tee-**ehn**-eh proh-**bleh**-mahs)
12. Diabetes?	¿Diabetes?	(**dee**-ah-beh-tehs)
13. Hypertension?	¿Presión alta?	(preh-see-**ohn ahl**-tah)
14. Heart disease?	¿Problemas de corazón?	(proh-**bleh**-mahs deh kohr-ah-**sohn**)
15. What medicines do you take?	¿Qué medicamentos toma?	(**keh** meh-dee-kah-**mehn**-tohs **toh**-mah)
16. Is there someone in your family with eye problems?	¿Hay alguien en su familia con problemas en la vista?	(eye ahl-gee-**ehn** en soo fah-mee-**lee**-ah kohn proh-**bleh**-mahs ehn lah **vees**-tah)
17. Is someone blind in your family?	¿Está alguien ciego en su familia?	(ehs-**tah** ahl-goo-**ehn** see-**eh**-goh ehn soo fah-mee-**lee**-ah)
18. From birth?	¿De nacimiento?	(deh nah-see-mee-**ehn**-toh)
19. When they became older?	¿Cuándo se hizo mayor?	(koo-**ahn**-doh seh **ee**-soh meye-**ohr**)
20. Do you wear glasses?	¿Usa anteojos?	(**oo**-sah ahn-teh-**oh**-hohs)
21. For reading?	¿Para leer?	(pah-rah leh-**ehr**)
22. For distances?	¿De lejos?	(deh **leh**-hohs)
23. Do you wear contact lenses?	¿Usa lentes de contacto?	(**oo**-sah **lehn**-tehs deh kohn-**tahk**-toh)
24. Hard?	¿Duros?	(**doo**-rohs)
25. Soft?	¿Blandos?	(**blahn**-dohs)

26. Do you take them out every night?	¿Se los quita todas las noches?	(seh lohs **kee**-tah toh-dahs lahs **noh**-chehs)

EYE EXAM

1. Please cover one eye	Por favor tápese un ojo	(pohr fah-vohr **tah**-peh-seh oon **oh**-hoh)
2. Read the letters on the board	Lea las letras en la pizarra	(leh-ah lahs **leh**-trahs ehn lah pee-**sahr**-ah)
3. Look through the pinholes	Mire a través de los agujeros	(**mee**-reh ah trah-**vehs** deh lohs ah-goo-**hehr**-ohs)
4. Can you see the letters better?	¿Puede ver las letras mejor?	(poo-**eh**-deh vehr lahs **leh**-trahs meh-**hohr**)
5. Cover the other eye	Cúbrase el otro ojo	(**koo**-brah-seh ehl **oh**-troh **oh**-hoh)
6. Follow my finger with your eyes	Siga mi dedo con su ojo	(**see**-gah mee **deh**-doh kohn soo **oh**-hoh)
7. Are you seeing double now?	¿Está viendo doble ahora?	(ehs-**tah** vee-**ehn**-doh **doh**-bleh ah-**ohr**-ah)
8. Cover one eye and look at my nose	Cúbrase un ojo y mire mi nariz	(**koo**-brah-seh oon **oh**-hoh ee mee-reh mee nhr-**ees**)
9. Keep looking at my nose and tell me how many fingers I am holding up?	¿Siga mirando mi nariz y dígame cuántos dedos ve?	(**see**-gah mee-**rahn**-doh mee nah-**rees** ee **dee**-gah-meh - koo-**ahn**-tohs **deh**-dohs veh)
10. Look straight ahead	Mire delante	(mee-reh deh-**lahn**-teh)
11. Look at the light at the end of the room	Mire la luz al fondo de la habitación	(mee-reh lah loos ahl **fohn**-doh deh lah ah-bee-tah-see-**ohn**)
12. Place your chin right here	Ponga su barbilla aquí	(**pohn**-gah soo bahr-**bee**-yah ah-**kee**)
13. Place your forehead up against the bar	Ponga su frente contra la barra	(**pohn**-gah soo **frehn**-teh kohn-trah lah **bah**-rah)

14. Look up	Mire arriba	(mee-reh ah-**ree**-bah)
15. Look down	Mire abajo	(mee-reh ah-**bah**-hoh)
16. Look right	Mire a la derecha	(mee-reh ah lah deh-**reh**-chah)
17. Look left	Mire a la izquierda	(mee-reh ah lah ees-kee-**ehr**-dah)
18. I am going to put a drop in your eye	Voy a poner una gota en su ojo	(voy ah pohn-**ehr** oon-ah **goh**-tah ehn soo **oh**-hoh)
19. Lean your head back	Ponga su cabeza hacia atrás	(**pohn**-gah soo kah-**beh**-sah ah-**see**-ah ah-**trahs**)
20. I am going to check the pressure in your eye	Voy a revisar la presión de su ojo	(voy ah re-vee-**sahr** lah preh-see-**ohn** deh soo **oh**-hoh)
21. I am going to put drops in your eyes that will dilate your pupils	Voy a ponerle unas gotas en sus ojos que dilatarán sus pupilas	(voy ah pohn-**ehr**-leh oon-ahs **goh**-tahs ehn soos **oh**-hoohs keh dee-lah-tahr-**ahn** soos poo-**pee**-lahs)
22. These drops will make your vision blurry for a few hours	Estas gotas harán su visión borrosa por unas horas	(ehs-tahs goh-tahs ah-**rahn** soo vee-see-**ohn** bohr-**oh**-sah pohr oon-ahs **ohr**-ahs)
23. These drops take a half an hour to work	Estas gotas tardan media hora en hacer efecto	(Ehs-tahs **goh**-tahs tahr-dahn meh-**dee**-ah **ohr**-ah ehn ah-**sehr** eh-**fehk**-toh)
24. I am going to have you wait out front until the drops have worked	Tiene que esperar fuera hasta que las gotas hagan efecto	(tee-**ehn**-eh keh ehs-pehr-**ahr** foo-**ehr**-ah **ahs**-tah keh lahs **goh**-tahs ah-gahn eh-**fehk**-toh)

HISTORY AND PHYSICAL

1. Do you have any problems with your eye?	¿Tiene algún problema con su ojo?	(tee-**eh**-neh ahl-**goon** proh-**bleh**-mah kohn soo **oh**-hoh)
2. Which eye?	¿Cuál ojo?	(koo-**ahl** **oh**-hoh)

3. Have you had this problem before?	¿Ha tenido usted este problema anteriormente?	(ah teh-**nee**-doh oos-**tehd** ehs-teh proh-**bleh**-mah ahn-tehr-ee-ohr-**mehn**-teh)
4. How long have you had this problem?	¿Desde cuándo tiene este problema?	(dehs-deh koo-**ahn**-doh tee-**eh**-neh ehs-teh proh-**bleh**-mah)
5. Days, weeks, months, years	Días, semanas, meses, años	(**dee**-ahs, seh-**mah**-nahs, **meh**-sehs, **ah**-nyohs)
6. Is your vision worse?	¿Está su vista peor?	(ehs-**tah** soo **vees**-tah peh-**ohr**)

APPENDICES
Section Ten

1. NUMBERS, DAYS, MONTHS, TIME

NUMBERS

0	Cero	(**seh**-roh)
1	Uno	(**oo**-noh)
2	Dos	(dohs)
3	Tres	(trehs)
4	Cuatro	(koo-**ah**-troh)
5	Cinco	(**seen**-koh)
6	Seis	(**seh**-ees)
7	Siete	(see-**eh**-teh)
8	Ocho	(**oh**-choh)
9	Nueve	(noo-**eh**-veh)
10	Diez	(dee-**ehs**)
11	Once	(**ohn**-seh)
12	Doce	(**doh**-seh)
13	Trece	(**treh**-seh)
14	Catorce	(kah-**tohr**-seh)
15	Quince	(**keen**-seh)
16	Dieciséis	(dee-ehs-ee-**seh**-ees)
17	Diecisiete	(dee-ehs-ee-see-**eh**-teh)
18	Dieciocho	(dee-ehs-ee-**oh**-choh)
19	Diecinueve	(dee-ehs-ee-noo-**eh**-beh)
20	Veinte	(veh-**een**-teh)
21	Veintiuno	(veh-een-tee-**oon**-oh)

30	Treinta	(treh-**ehn**-tah)
40	Cuarenta	(koo-ahr-**ehn**-tah)
50	Cincuenta	(seen-koo-**ehn**-tah)
60	Sesenta	(seh-**sehn**-teh)
70	Setenta	(seh-**tehn**-tah)
80	Ochenta	(oh-**chen**-tah)
90	Noventa	(noh-**behn**-tah)
100	Cien	(**see**-ehn)
100.5	Ciento punto cinco	(see-**ehn**-toh **poon**-toh **seen**-koh)
100.7	Ciento punto siete	(see-**ehn**-toh **poon**-toh see-**eh**-teh)
101	Ciento uno	(see-**ehn**-toh **oo**-noh)
102	Ciento dos	(see-**ehn**-toh dohs)

DAYS OF THE WEEK

1. Sunday	Domingo	(doh-**meen**-goh)
2. Monday	Lunes	(**loo**-nehs)
3. Tuesday	Martes	(**mahr**-tehs)
4. Wednesday	Miércoles	(mee-**ehr**-koh-lehs)
5. Thursday	Jueves	(hoo-**eh**-behs)
6. Friday	Viernes	(vee-**ehr**-nehs)
7. Saturday	Sábado	(**sah**-bah-doh)

MONTHS OF THE YEAR

1. January	Enero	(eh-**neh**-roh)
2. February	Febrero	(feh-**breh**-roh)

3. March	Marzo	(**mahr**-soh)
4. April	Abril	(ah-**breel**)
5. May	Mayo	(**mah**-yoh)
6. June	Junio	(hoo-**nee**-oh)
7. July	Julio	(hoo-**lee**-oh)
8. August	Agosto	(ah-**gohs**-toh)
9. September	Septiembre	(sehp-tee-**ehm**-breh)
10. October	Octubre	(ohk-**too**-breh)
11. November	Noviembre	(noh-vee-**ehm**-breh)
12. December	Diciembre	(dee-see-**ehm**-breh)

TIME

1. Now	Ahora	(ah-**oh**-rah)
2. Today	Hoy	(oy)
3. Yesterday	Ayer	(eye-**ehr**)
4. Day before yesterday	Anteayer	(ahn-teh-eye-**ehr**)
5. In the morning	En la mañana	(ehn lah mah-**nyah**-nah)
6. In the afternoon	En la tarde	(ehn lah **tahr**-deh)
7. In the evening	En la noche	(ehn lah **noh**-cheh)
8. Seconds	Segundos	(seh-**goon**-dohs)
9. Minutes	Minutos	(meen-**oo**-tohs)
10. Hours	Horas	(**ohr**-ahs)
11. Days	Días	(**dee**-ahs)
12. Weeks	Semanas	(seh-**mah**-nahs)
13. Months	Meses	(**meh**-sehs)
14. Years	Años	(**ah**-nyohs)

2. FAMILY VOCABULARY

1. Father	Padre	(**pah**-dreh)
2. Mother	Madre	(**mah**-dreh)
3. Sister	Hermana	(ehr-**mah**-nah)
4. Brother	Hermano	(ehr-**mah**-noh)
5. Wife	Esposa	(ehs-**poh**-sah)
6. Husband	Esposo	(ehs-**poh**-soh)
7. Son	Hijo	(**ee**-hoh)
8. Daughter	Hija	(**ee**-hah)
9. Baby	Bebé	(beh-**beh**)
10. Relative	Pariente	(pah-ree-**ehn**-teh)
11. Cousin	Primo	(**pree**-moh)
12. Aunt	Tía	(**tee**-ah)
13. Uncle	Tío	(**tee**-oh)
14. Nephew	Sobrino	(soh-**bree**-noh)
15. Niece	Sobrina	(soh-**bree**-nah)
16. Boyfriend	Novio	(noh-**vee**-oh)
17. Girlfriend	Novia	(noh-**vee**-ah)

3. COLORS

1. Red	Rojo	(**roh**-hoh)
2. Yellow	Amarillo	(ah-mah-**ree**-yoh)

3. Green	Verde	(**behr**-deh)
4. Gray	Gris	(grees)
5. Black	Negro	(**neh**-groh)
6. Dark	Obscuro	(ohs-**koo**-roh)
7. Clear	Claro	(**klah**-roh)
8. White	Blanco	(**blahn**-koh)

4. ANATOMY VOCABULARY

CHAPTER OUTLINE

HEAD AND NECK (EXTRACRANIAL)

1. Hair	El pelo	(ehl **peh**-loh)
2. Scalp	Cuero cabelludo	(koo-**eh**-roh kah-beh-**yoo**-doh)
3. Skull	El cráneo	(ehl **krah**-neh-oh)
4. Forehead	La frente	(lah **frehn**-teh)

5. Head	La cabeza	(lah kah-**beh**-sah)
6. Eyes	Los ojos	(lohs **oh**-hohs)
7. Eyelashes	Las pestañas	(lahs pehs-**tah**-nahs)
8. Eyelids	Los párpados	(lohs **pahr**-pah-dohs)
9. Face	La cara	(lah **kah**-rah)
10. Ears	Los oídos	(lohs oh-**ee**-dohs)
11. Nose	La nariz	(lah nahr-**ees**)
12. Nasal bone	El hueso nasal	(ehl oo-**eh**-soh nahs-**ahl**)
13. Mouth	La boca	(lah **boh**-kah)
14. Lips	Los labios	(lohs **lah**-bee-ohs)
15. Tongue	La lengua	(lah **lehn**-goo-ah)
16. Teeth	Los dientes	(lohs dee-**ehn**-tehs)
17. Tonsils	Las amígdalas	(lahs ah-**meeg**-dah-lahs)
18. Throat	La garganta	(lah gahr-**gahn**-tah)
19. Jaw	La mandíbula	(lah mahn-**dee**-boo-lah)
20. Chin	La barbilla	(lah bahr-**bee**-yah)
21. Neck	El cuello	(ehl koo-**eh**-yoh)
22. Lymph nodes	Los nódulos linfáticos	(los **noh**-doo-lohs leen-**fah**-tee-kohs)
23. Thyroid	La tiroide	(lah teer-**oy**-deh)

INTRACRANIAL

1. Central nervous system	El sistema nervioso central	(ehl sees-**teh**-mah nehr-vee-**oh**-soh sehn-**trahl**)
2. Brain	El cerebro	(ehl sehr-**eh**-broh)

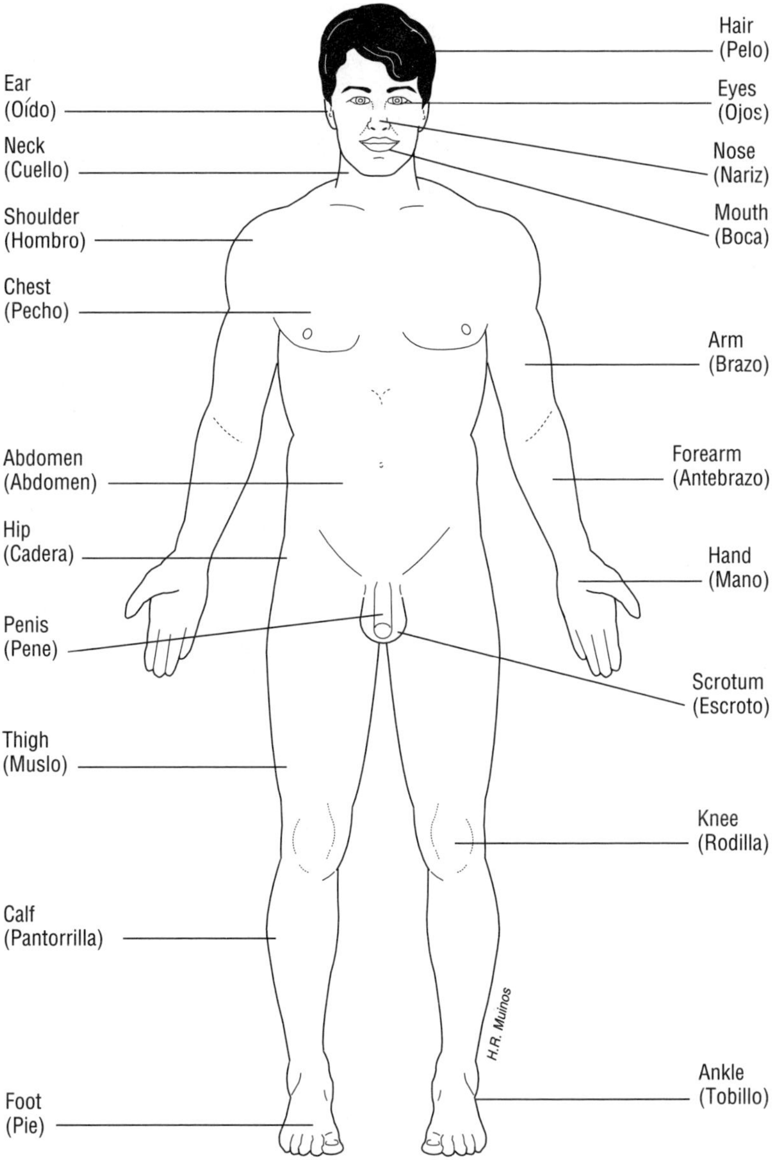

Figure 4. Adult male (front view).

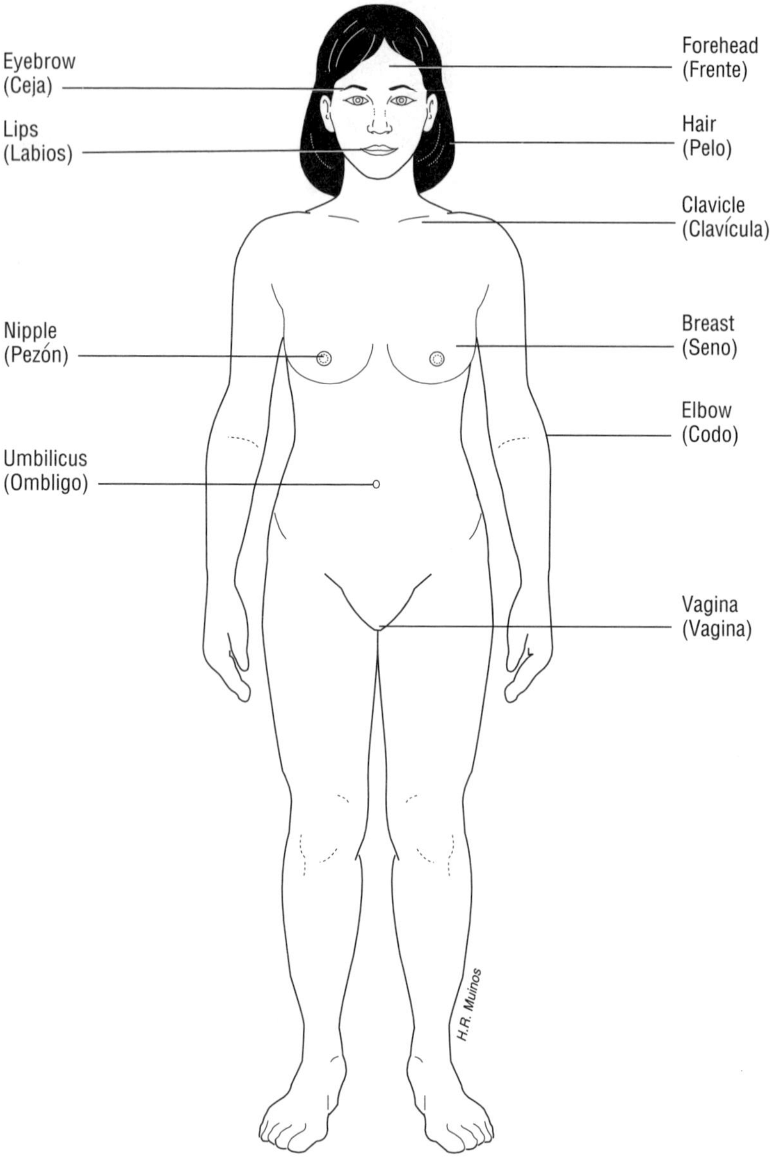

Figure 5. Adult female (front view).

3. Frontal lobe	Lóbulo frontal	(**loh**-boo-loh frohn-**tahl**)
4. Temporal lobe	Lóbulo temporal	(**loh**-boo-loh tehm-pohr-**ahl**)
5. Parietal lobe	Lóbulo parietal	(**loh**-boo-loh pahr-ee-eh-**tahl**)
6. Occipital lobe	Lóbulo occipital	(**loh**-boo-loh oh-see-pee-**tahl**)
7. Basal ganglia	Los ganglios basales	(lohs **gahn**-glee-ohs bah-**sahl**-ehs)
8. Corpus callosum	Cuerpo calloso	(**kohr**-poo kah-**loh**-soh)
9. Lateral ventricle	El ventrículo lateral	(ehl vehn-**tree**-koo-loh lah-tehr-**ahl**)
10. Choroid plexus	El plexo coroide	(ehl **plehx**-oh kohr-**oy**-deh)
11. Third ventricle	El tercer ventrículo	(ehl tehr-**sehr** vehn-**tree**-koo-loh)

ARTERIES OF THE HEAD AND NECK

1. Brachiocephalic artery	La arteria braquiocefálica	(Lah ahr-tehr-**ee**-ah brah-kee-oh-seh-**fahl**-ee-kah)
2. Common carotid artery	La arteria carótida común	(lah ahr-tehr-**ee**-ah kahr-**oh**-tee-dah koh-**moon**)
3. Internal carotid	Carótida interna	(cahr-**oh**-tee-dah een-**tehr**-nah)
4. External carotid	Carótida externa	(kahr-**oh**-tee-dah ehx-**tehr**-nah)
5. Intracranial segment	El segmento intracraneal	(ehl sehg-**mehn**-toh een-trah-krahn-ee-**ahl**)
6. Anterior cerebral artery	La arteria cerebral anterior	(lah ahr-tehr-**ee**-ah seh-reh-**brahl** ahn-tehr-ee-**ohr**)
7. Middle cerebral artery	La arteria cerebral media	(lah ahr-tehr-**ee**-ah seh-reh-**brahl** meh-**dee**-ah)

8. Posterior cerebral artery	La arteria cerebral posterior	(lah ahr-tehr-**ee**-ah seh-reh-**brahl** pohs-tehr-ee-**ohr**)
9. Vertebral artery	La arteria vertebral	(lah ahr-tehr-**ee**-ah vehr-teh-**brahl**)
10. Basilar artery	La arteria basilar	(lah ahr-tehr-**ee**-ah bah-see-**lahr**)

VEINS OF THE HEAD AND NECK

1. Superficial veins	Venas superficiales	(**veh**-nahs soo-pehr-fee-see-**ahl**-ehs)
2. Deep veins	Venas profundas	(**veh**-nahs proh-**foon**-dahs)
3. Vein of Galen	Vena de Galeno	(**veh**-nah deh gah-**leh**-noh)
4. Superior sagittal sinus	El seno sagital superior	(ehl **seh**-noh sah-hee-**tahl** soo-pehr-ee-**ohr**)
5. Internal jugular vein	Vena yugular interna	(**veh**-nah yoo-goo-**lahr** een-**tehr**-nah)
6. External jugular vein	Vena yugular externa	(**veh**-nah yoo-goo-**lahr** ehx-**tehr**-nah)

LUNGS

1. Right lung	El pulmón derecho	(ehl pool-**mohn** deh-**reh**-choh)
2. Upper lobe	Lóbulo superior	(**loh**-boo-loh soo-pehr-ee-**ohr**)
3. Middle lobe	Lóbulo medio	(**loh**-boo-loh meh-**dee**-oh)
4. Lower lobe	Lóbulo inferior	(**loh**-boo-loh een-fehr-ee-**ohr**)
5. Pleural space	Espacio pleural	(ehs-**pah**-see-oh pleh-oo-**rahl**)
6. Trachea	Tráquea	(**trah**-keh-ah)

7. Bronchus	Bronquio	(brohn-**kee**-oh)
8. Carina	Carina	(kahr-**ee**-nah)
9. Mediastinum	Mediastino	(meh-dee-ah-**stee**-noh)
10. Diaphragm	El diafragma	(ehl dee-ah-**frahg**-mah)
11. Chest	El pecho	(ehl **peh**-choh)
12. Breast	El pecho o el seno	(ehl **peh**-choh oh ehl **seh**-noh)
13. Nipple	El pezón	(ehl peh-**sohn**)
14. Ribs	Las costillas	(lahs kohs-**tee**-yahs)
15. Sternum	Esternón	(ehs-ter-**nohn**)
16. Manubrium	Manubrium	(mah-**noo**-bree-oom)
17. Clavicle	La clavícula	(lah klah-**vee**-koo-lah)
18. Scapula	Escápula	(ehs-**kah**-poo-lah)

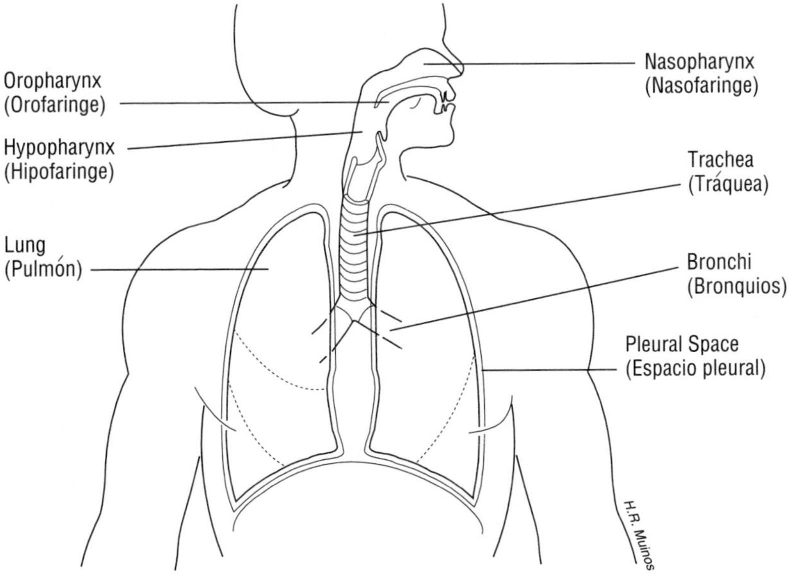

Figure 6. The respiratory system.

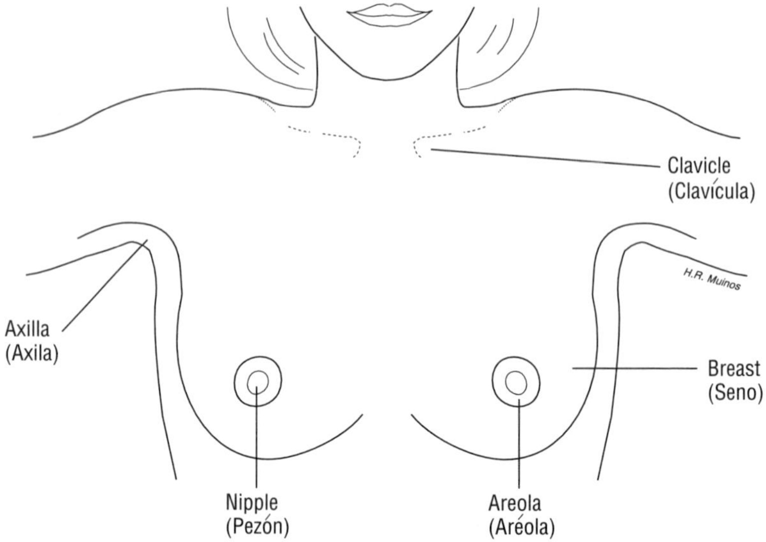

Figure 7. The female breast.

ARTERIES AND VEINS OF THORAX

1. Aortic root	La raíz de la aorta	(lah rah-**ees** deh lah ah-**ohr**-tah)
2. Ascending aorta	Aorta ascendente	(ah-**ohr**-tah ah-sehn-**dehn**-teh)
3. Aortic arch	El arco aórtico	(ehl **ahr**-koh ah-**ohr**-tee-koh)
4. Aortic knob	Botón aórtico	(boh-**tohn** ah-**ohr**-tee-koh)
5. Descending aorta	Aorta descendente	(ah-**ohr**-tah deh-sehn-**dehn**-teh)
6. Subclavian artery	La arteria subclavia	(lah ahr-tehr-**ee**-ah soob-klah-**vee**-ah)
7. Superior vena cava	Vena cava superior	(**veh**-nah **kah**-vah soo-pehr-ee-**ohr**)
8. Brachiocephalic vein	Vena braquiocefálica	(**veh**-nah brah-kee-oh-seh-**fah**-lee-kah)
9. Subclavian vein	Vena subclavia	(**veh**-nah soob-klah-**vee**-ah)

HEART

1.	Right atrium	Aurícula derecha	(ah-oo-**ree**-koo-lah deh-**reh**-chah)
2.	Right ventricle	Ventrículo derecho	(vehn-**tree**-koo-loh deh-**reh**-choh)
3.	Ventricular septum	Tabique ventricular	(tah-**bee**-keh vehn-tree-koo-**lahr**)
4.	Main pulmonary artery	Arteria pulmonar principal	(ahr-tehr-**ee**-ah pool-mohn-**ahr** preen-see-**pahl**)
5.	Pulmonary veins	Venas pulmonares	(**veh**-nahs pool-mohn-**ahr**-ehs)
6.	Left atrium	Aurícula izquierda	(ah-oo-**ree**-koo-lah ees-kee-**ehr**-doh)
7.	Left ventricle	Ventrículo izquierdo	(vehn-**tree**-koo-loh ees-kee-**ehr**-doh)
8.	Tricuspid valve	Válvula tricúspide	(**vahl**-voo-lah tree-**koos**-pee-deh)
9.	Pulmonary valve	Válvula pulmonar	(**vahl**-voo-lah pool-mohn-**ahr**)
10.	Mitral valve	Válvula mitral	(**vahl**-voo-lah mee-**trahl**)
11.	Aortic valve	Válvula aórtica	(**vahl**-voo-lah ah-**ohr**-tee-kah)
12.	Chordae tendinae	Cuerda tendinea	(koo-**ehr**-dah tehn-**deen**-eh-ah)
13.	Papillary muscles	Músculos papilares	(**moos**-koo-lohs pah-pee-**lahr**-ehs)
14.	Apex	El ápice	(ehl **ah**-pee-seh)
15.	Cardiac silhouette	La silueta cardíaca	(lah see-loo-**eh**-tah kahr-**dee**-ah-kah)
16.	Right coronary artery	Arteria coronaria derecha	(ahr-tehr-**ee**-ah kohr-ohn-ahr-**ee**-ah deh-**reh**-chah)
17.	Pericardium	Pericardio	(pehr-ee-kahr-**dee**-oh)

GASTROINTESTINAL TRACT (GIT)

1. Esophagus	El esófago	(ehl eh-**soh**-fah-goh)
2. Stomach	El estómago	(ehl eh-**stoh**-mah-goh)
3. Fundus	Fundo	(**foon**-doh)
4. Body	Cuerpo	(koo-**ehr**-poh)
5. Antrum	Antro	(**ahn**-troh)
6. Pylorus	Píloro	(**pee**-lohr-oh)
7. Gastric folds	Pliegues gástricos	(plee-eh-gehs **gahs**-tree-kohs)
8. Duodenum	El duodeno	(ehl doo-oh-**deh**-noh)
9. Jejunum	Yeyuno	(yeh-**yoo**-noh)
10. Ileum	Ileón	(eel-eh-**ohn**)
11. Terminal ileum	Ileo terminal	(eel-**eh**-oh tehr-mee-**nahl**)
12. Small intestine	Intestino delgado	(een-tehs-**tee**-noh dehl-**gah**-doh)
13. Bowel gas	Gases intestinales	(**gah**-sehs een-tehs-tee-**nah**-lehs)
14. Appendix	El apéndice	(ehl ah-**pehn**-dee-seh)
15. Cecum	Ciego	(see-**eh**-goh)
16. Large intestine	Intestino grueso	(een-tehs-**tee**-noh groo-**ehs**-oh)
17. Colon	El colon	(ehl **koh**-lohn)
18. Ascending colon	Colon ascendente	(**koh**-lohn ahs-sehn-**dehn**-teh)
19. Hepatic flexure	Ángulo hepático	(**ahn**-goo-loh eh-**pah**-tee-koh)
20. Transverse colon	Colon transverso	(**koh**-lohn trahns-**vehr**-soh)
21. Splenic flexure	Ángulo esplénico	(**ahn**-goo-loh ehs-**pleh**-nee-koh)
22. Descending colon	Colon descendente	(**koh**-lohn dehs-sehn-**dehn**-teh)

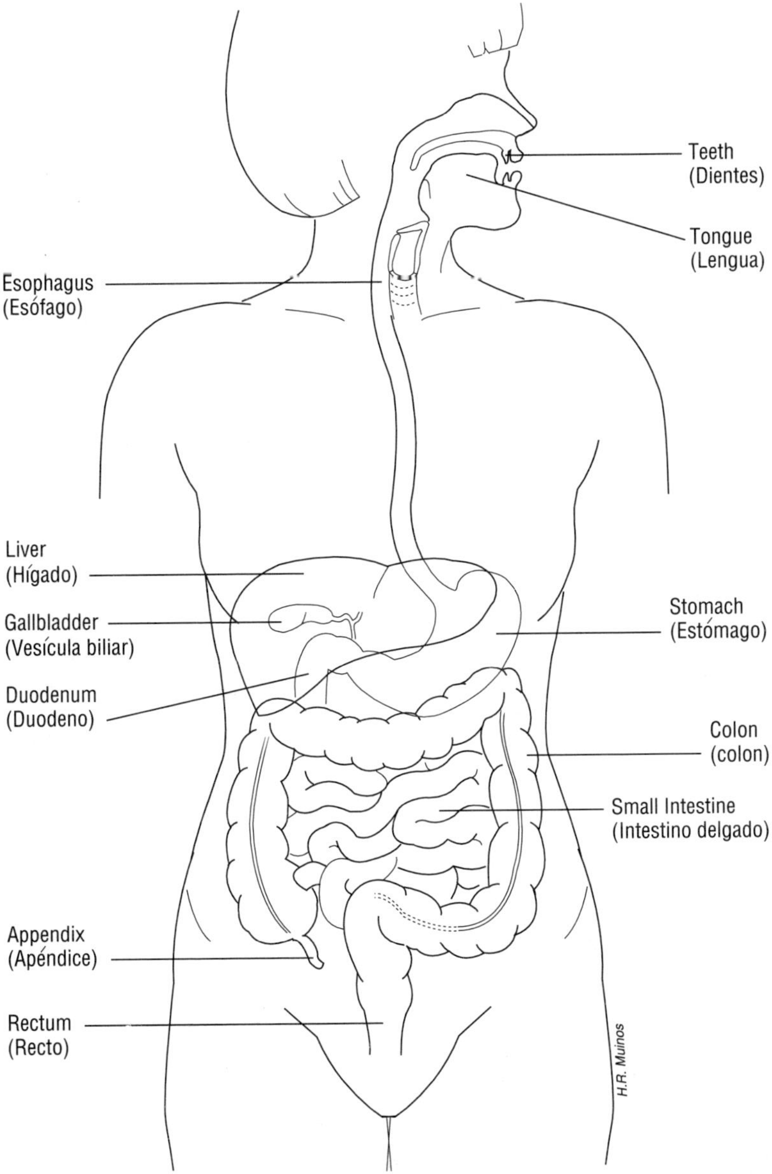

Figure 8. The digestive system.

23. Sigmoid	Sigmoide	(seeg-**moy**-deh)
24. Rectum	Recto	(**rehk**-toh)
25. Anus	Ano	(**ah**-noh)

SOLID ORGANS OF THE ABDOMEN AND RELATED STRUCTURES

1. Liver	El hígado	(ehl **ee**-gah-doh)
2. Spleen	El bazo	(ehl **bah**-soh)
3. Pancreas	El páncreas	(ehl **pahn**-kreh-ahs)
4. Adrenal gland	Glándula adrenal	(**glahn**-doo-lah ah-dreh-**nahl**)
5. Kidney	El riñón	(ehl ree-**nyohn**)
6. Gallbladder	La vesícula biliar	(lah veh-**see**-koo-lah bee-lee-**ahr**)

ARTERIES AND VEINS OF THE ABDOMEN

1. Abdominal aorta	Aorta abdominal	(ah-**ohr**-tah ahb-doh-mee-**nahl**)
2. Celiac artery	Arteria celíaca	(ahr-tehr-**ee**-ah seh-**lee**-ah-kah)
3. Hepatic artery	Arteria hepática	(ahr-tehr-**ee**-ah eh-**pah**-tee-kah)
4. Splenic artery	Arteria esplénica	(ahr-tehr-**ee**-ah ehs-**pleh**-nee-kah)
5. Superior mesenteric artery	Arteria mesentérica superior	(ahr-tehr-**ee**-ah mehs-ehn-**tehr**-ee-kah soo-pehr-ee-**ohr**)
6. Renal artery	Arteria renal	(ahr-tehr-**ee**-ah reh-**nahl**)
7. Inferior mesenteric artery	Arteria mesentérica inferior	(ahr-tehr-**ee**-ah mehs-ehn-**tehr**-ee-kah een-fehr-ee-**ohr**)
8. Inferior vena cava	Vena cava inferior	(**veh**-nah **kah**-vah een-fehr-ee-**ohr**)

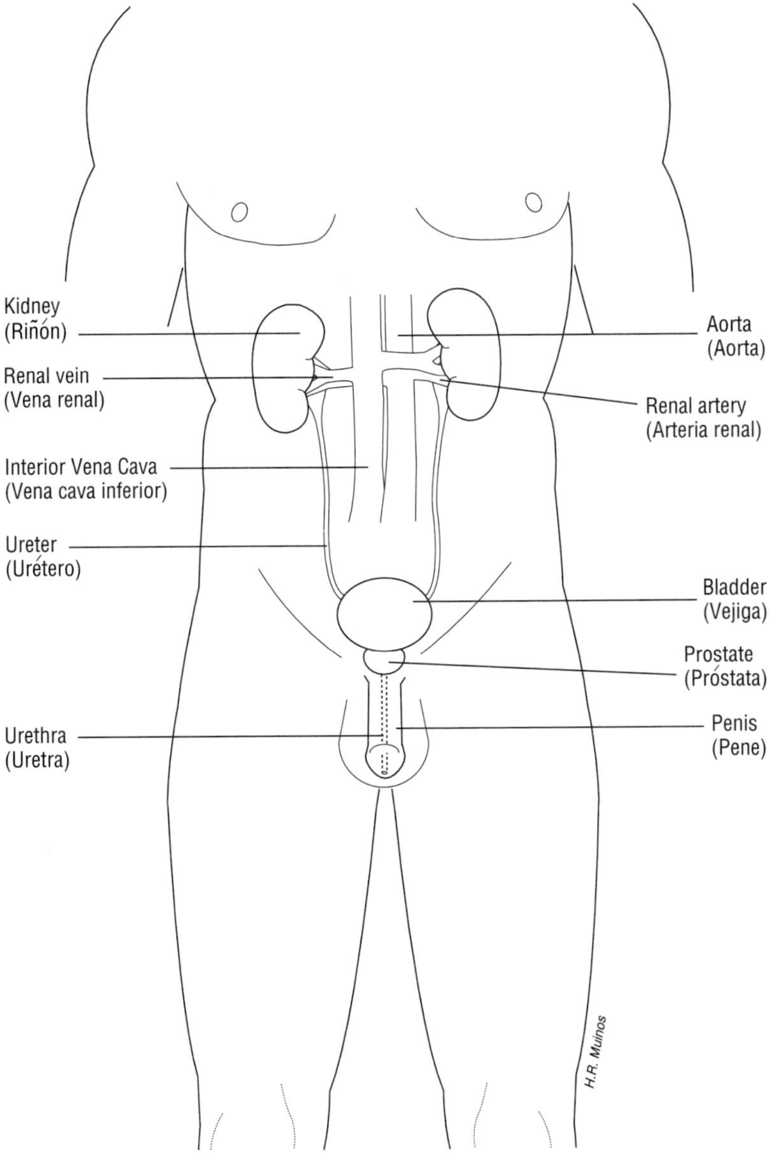

Figure 9. The urinary tract (male).

9. Renal vein	Vena renal	(**veh**-nah reh-**nahl**)
10. Portal vein	Vena portal	(**veh**-nah pohr-**tahl**)

PELVIS

1. Ovary	Ovario	(oh-**vahr**-ee-oh)
2. Follicle	Folículo	(foh-**lee**-koo-loh)
3. Corpus luteum	Cuerpo lúteo	(koo-**ehr**-poh **loo**-teh-oh)
4. Fallopian tube	Trompas de Falopio	(**trohm**-pahs deh fal-**loh**-pee-oh)
5. Uterus	El útero o la matriz	(ehl **oo**-tehr-oh oh lah mah-**trees**)
6. Cervix	La cerviz o el cuello de la matriz	(lah sehr-**vees** oh ehl koo-**eh**-yoh deh lah mah-**trees**)
7. Vagina	La vagina	(lah vah-**hee**-nah)

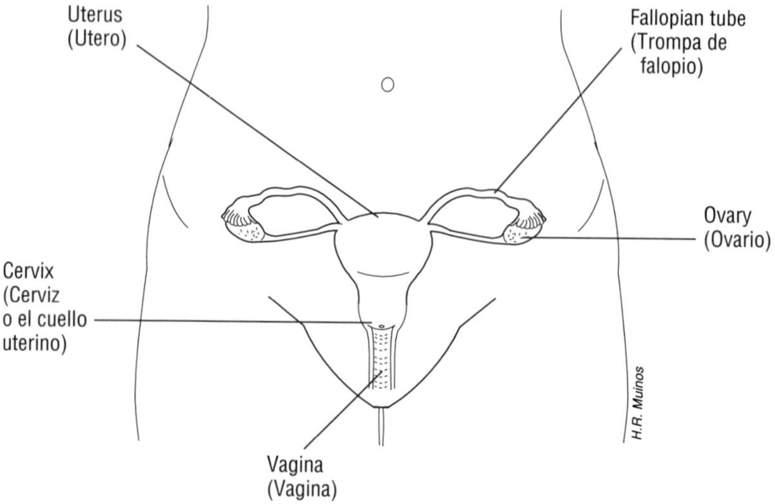

Figure 10. The female reproductive system.

8. Scrotum	El escroto	(ehl ehs-**croh**-toh)
9. Testicles	Los testículos	(lohs tehs-**tee**-koo-lohs)
10. Prostate	La próstata	(lah **prohs**-tah-tah)
11. Penis	El pene	(ehl **peh**-neh)
12. Bladder	La vejiga	(lah veh-**hee**-gah)
13. Sacrum	Sacro	(**sah**-kroh)
14. Pubic symphysis	Sínfisis púbica	(**seen**-fee-sees **poo**-bee-kah)
15. Waist	La cintura	(lah seen-**too**-rah)

BACK

1. Back	La espalda	(lah ehs-**pahl**-dah)
2. Vertical column	La columna vertebral	(lah koh-**loom**-nah vehr-tah-**brahl**)
3. Spine	Espina	(ehs-**pee**-nah)
4. Vertebra	Vértebra	(**vehr**-teh-brah)
5. Spinal cord	Médula espinal	(**meh**-doo-lah ehs-pee-**nahl**)

UPPER EXTREMITY

1. Shoulder	Hombro	(**ohm**-broh)
2. Humerus	Húmero	(**oom**-ehr-oh)
3. Elbow	El codo	(ehl **koh**-doh)
4. Radius	Radio	(rah-**dee**-oh)
5. Ulna	Cúbito	(**koo**-bee-toh)
6. Wrist	La muñeca	(lah moo-**nyeh**-kah)
7. Hand	La mano	(lah **mah**-noh)
8. Fingers	Los dedos	(lohs **deh**-dohs)

9. Thumb	El pulgar	(ehl pool-**gahr**)
10. Index finger	Dedo índice	(**deh**-doh **een**-dee-seh)
11. Middle finger	Dedo del corazón o dedo medio	(**deh**-doh dehl kohr-ah-**sohn** oh **deh**-doh meh-**dee**-oh)
12. Ring finger	Dedo anular	(**deh**-doh ah-noo-**lahr**)
13. Little finger	Dedo pequeño o dedo meñique	(**deh**-doh peh-**keh**-nyoh oh **deh**-doh meh-**nee**-keh)
14. Axillary artery	Arteria axilar	(ahr-tehr-**ee**-ah ahx-ee-**lahr**)
15. Brachial artery	Arteria braquial	(ahr-tehr-**ee**-ah brah-kee-**ahl**)
16. Radial artery	Arteria radial	(ahr-tehr-**ee**-ah rah-dee-**ahl**)
17. Ulnar artery	Arteria ulnar	(ahr-tehr-**ee**-ah ool-**nahr**)
18. Basilic vein	Vena basílica	(**veh**-nah bah-**see**-lee-kah)
19. Cephalic vein	Vena cefálica	(**veh**-nah seh-**fahl**-ee-kah)
20. Axillary vein	Vena axilar	(**veh**-nah ahx-ee-**lahr**)

LOWER EXTREMITY

1. Hip	La cadera	(lah kah-**dehr**-ah)
2. Acetabulum	Acetábulo	(ah-seh-**tah**-boo-loh)
3. Femur	Fémur	(**feh**-moor)
4. Femoral head	Cabeza femoral o cabeza del fémur	(kah-**beh**-sah feh-mohr-**ahl** oh kah-**beh**-sah dehl **feh**-moor)
5. Knee	La rodilla	(lah roh-**dee**-yah)
6. Tibia	La tibia	(lah tee-**bee**-ah)
7. Fibula	Peroné	(pehr-ohn-**eh**)
8. Ankle	El tobillo	(ehl toh-**bee**-yoh)
9. Foot	El pie	(ehl **pee**-eh)

10. Toes	Los dedos del pie	(lohs **deh**-dohs dehl **pee**-eh)
11. Common iliac artery	Arteria ilíaca común	(ahr-tehr-**ee**-ah ee-**lee**-ah-kah koh-**moon**)
12. External iliac artery	Arteria ilíaca externa	(ahr-tehr-**ee**-ah ee-**lee**-ah-kah ehx-**tehr**-nah)
13. Common femoral artery	Arteria femoral común	(ahr-tehr-**ee**-ah feh-mohr-**ahl** koh-**moon**)
14. Superficial femoral artery	Arteria femoral superficial	(ahr-tehr-**ee**-ah feh-mohr-**ahl** soo-pehr-fee-see-**ahl**)
15. Deep femoral artery	Arterial femoral profunda	(ahr-tehr-ee-**ahl** feh-moor-**ahl** proh-**foon**-dah)
16. Popliteal artery	Arteria poplítea	(ahr-tehr-**ee**-ah poh-**plee**-teh-ah)
17. Anterior tibial artery	Arteria tibial anterior	(ahr-tehr-**ee**-ah tee-bee-**ahl** ahn-tehr-ee-**ohr**)
18. Posterior tibial artery	Arteria tibial posterior	(ahr-tehr-**ee**-ah tee-bee-**ahl** pohs-tehr-ee-**ohr**)
19. Common femoral vein	Vena femoral común	(**veh**-nah feh-mohr-**ahl** koh-**moon**)
20. Superficial femoral vein	Vena femoral superficial	(**veh**-nah feh-mohr-**ahl** soo-pehr-fee-see-**ahl**)
21. Popliteal vein	Vena poplítea	(**veh**-nah poh-**plee**-teh-ah)

MISCELLANEOUS

1. Skin	Piel	(pee-**ehl**)
2. Bone	El hueso	(ehl oo-**ehs**-soh)
3. Tendon	Tendón	(tehn-**dohn**)
4. Ligament	Ligamento	(lee-gah-**mehn**-toh)

5. Joint	Articulación	(ahr-tee-koo-lah-see-**ohn**)
6. Tissue	Tejido	(teh-**hee**-doh)
7. Muscle	Músculo	(**moos**-koo-loh)
8. Blood	La sangre	(lah **sahn**-greh)
9. Lymph	Linfa	(**leen**-fah)
10. Lymph nodes	Nódulos linfáticos	(**noh**-doo-lohs leen-**fah**-tee-kohs)
11. The body	El cuerpo	(ehl koo-**ehr**-poh)
12. Artery	Arteria	(ahr-tehr-**ee**-ah)
13. Arteriole	Arteriolas	(ahr-tehr-ee-**oh**-lahs)
14. Capillaries	Capilares	(ka-pee-**lahr**-ehs)
15. Fat tissue	Tejido grasoso	(teh-**hee**-doh grah-**soh**-soh)

5. ITEMS OF CLOTHING

1. Cap	Una gorra	(oon-ah **gohr**-ah)
2. Mask	Cubreboca o máscara	(koo-breh-**boh**-kah oh mahs-**kahr**-ah)
3. Gown	Bata	(**bah**-tah)
4. Glasses	Anteojos	(ahn-teh-**oh**-hohs)
5. Dentures	Dentaduras	(dehn-tah-**door**-ahs)
6. Shirt	Camisa	(kah-**mee**-sah)
7. Blouse	Blusa	(**bloo**-sah)
8. Pants	Pantalónes	(pahn-tah-**lohn**-ehs)

9. Dress	Un vestido	(oon vehs-**tee**-doh)
10. Underwear	Ropa interior	(**roh**-pah een-tehr-ee-**ohr**)
11. Socks	Los calcetines	(los kahl-seh-**tee**-nehs)
12. Shoes	Los zapatos	(lohs sah-**pah**-tohs)
13. Slippers	Las zapatillas	(lahs sah-pah-**tee**-yahs)
14. Boots	Las botas	(lahs **boh**-tahs)
15. Jacket	La chaqueta	(lah chah-**keh**-tah)
16. Gloves	Los guantes	(lohs goo-**ahn**-tehs)

6. USEFUL VERBS IN COMMAND FORM

1. Stand up	Párese	(**pahr**-ehs-eh)
2. Sit down	Siéntese	(see-**ehn**-teh-seh)
3. Lie down	Acuéstese	(ah-koo-**ehs**-teh-seh)
4. Lie on your back	Acuéstese boca arriba	(ah-koo-**ehs**-teh-seh **boh**-kah ah-**ree**-bah)
5. Turn onto your stomach	Colóquese boca bajo	(kohl-**loh**-keh-seh **boh**-kah **bah**-hoh)
6. Put your hand at your side	Ponga la mano a su lado	(**pohn**-gah lah **mah**-noh ah soo **lah**-doh)
7. Breathe	Respire	(rehs-**pee**-reh)
8. Do not breathe	No respire	(noh res-**pee**-reh)
9. Take a deep breath and hold it	Respire profundo y aguante	(rehs-**pee**-reh proh-**foon**-doh ee ah-goo-**ahn**-teh)

10. Push	Puje	(**poo**-heh)
11. Stop	Párese	(**pah**-reh-seh)
12. Do not push	No puje	(noh **poo**-heh)
13. Do this	Haga esto	(**ah**-gah **ehs**-toh)
14. Do not move	No se mueva	(noh seh moo-**eh**-vah)
15. Cough	Tosa	(**toh**-sah)
16. Come with me	Venga conmigo	(**vehn**-gah kohn-**mee**-goh)
17. Drink	Tome	(**toh**-meh)
18. Swallow	Trague	(**trah**-geh)
19. Squeeze my hand	Apriete mi mano	(ah-pree-**eh**-teh mee **mah**-noh)
20. Make a fist	Haga un puño	(**ah**-gah oon poo-**nyoh**)

7. THE PATIENT'S ROOM

1. Pillow	Almohada	(ahl-moh-**ah**-dah)
2. Blanket	Manta	(**mahn**-tah)
3. Bed	Cama	(**kah**-mah)
4. Table	Mesa	(**meh**-sah)
5. Telephone	Teléfono	(teh-**leh**-foh-noh)
6. Television	Televisión	(teh-leh-vee-see-**ohn**)
7. Controls for the television	Los controles del televisión	(lohs kohn-**troh**-lehs dehl teh-lah-vee-see-**ohn**)
8. On	Encendido	(ehn-sehn-**dee**-doh)

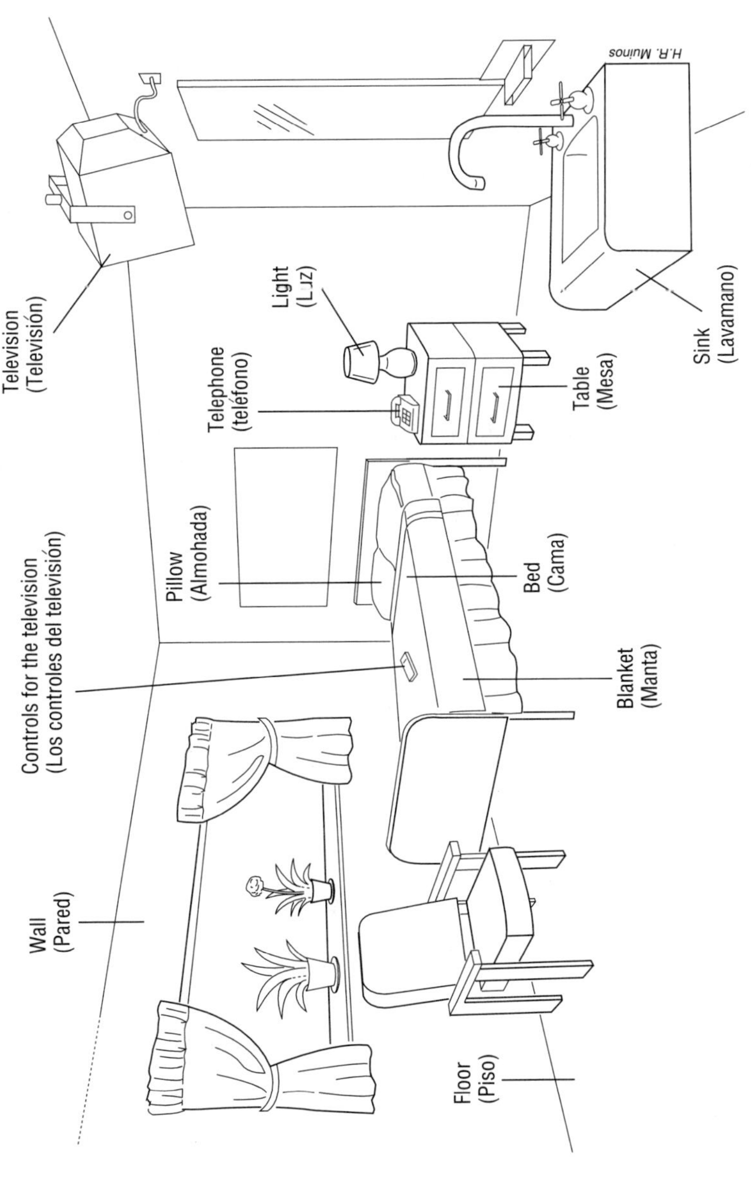

Figure 11. Hospital room.

APPENDICES

9.	Off	Apagado	(ah-pah-**gah**-doh)
10.	Volume	Volumen	(voh-**loo**-mehn)
11.	Button	Botón	(boh-**tohn**)
12.	Push this to call the nurse	Toque esto para llamar a la enfermera	(toh-keh ehs-toh pahr-ah **yah**-mahr ah lah ehn-fehr-**mehr**-ah)
13.	Bathroom	Baño	(**bah**-nyoh)
14.	Curtain	Cortina	(kohr-**tee**-nah)
15.	Door	Puerta	(poo-**ehr**-tah)
16.	Do you want it open or closed?	¿Quiere la puerta abierta o cerrada?	(kee-**ehr**-eh la poo-**ehr**-tah ah-bee-**ehr**-tah oh sehr-**ah**-dah)
17.	Open	Abierto	(ah-bee-**ehr**-toh)
18.	Closed	Cerrado	(sehr-**ah**-doh)

8. WORDS OF POSITION AND COMPARISON

1.	Open	Abierto	(ah-bee-**ehr**-toh)
2.	Closed	Cerrado	(sehr-**ah**-doh)
3.	Vacant	Libre	(**lee**-breh)
4.	Occupied	Ocupado	(oh-koo-**pah**-doh)
5.	More than	Más que	(**mahs** keh)
6.	Less than	Menos que	(**meh**-nohs keh)
7.	Fast	Rápido	(**rah**-pee-doh)
8.	Slow	Lento	(**lehn**-toh)
9.	Heavy	Pesado	(peh-**sah**-doh)

10. Light	Ligero	(lee-**gehr**-oh)
11. Young	Joven	(**hoh**-vehn)
12. Old	Viejo	(vee-**eh**-hoh)
13. Early	Temprano	(tehm-**prah**-noh)
14. Late	Tarde	(**tahr**-deh)
15. Easy	Fácil	(**fah**-seel)
16. Difficult	Difícil	(dee-**fee**-seel)
17. Full	Lleno	(**yeh**-noh)
18. Empty	Vacío	(vah-**see**-oh)
19. Next	El próximo	(ehl **prohx**-ee-moh)
20. Last	El último	(ehl **ool**-tee-moh)
21. Inside	Dentro	(**dehn**-troh)
22. Outside	Fuera	(foo-**ehr**-ah)
23. Central	Central	(sehn-**trahl**)
24. Peripheral	Periférico	(pehr-ee-**fehr**-ee-koh)
25. Diameter	Diámetro	(dee-**ah**-meh-troh)
26. Size	Tamaño	(tah-**mah**-nyoh)
27. Small	Pequeño	(peh-**keh**-nyoh)
28. Large	Grande	(**grahn**-deh)
29. Common	Común	(koh-**moon**)
30. Rare	Raro	(**rahr**-oh)
31. Hot	Caliente	(kah-lee-**ehn**-teh)
32. Cold	Frío	(**fee**-oh)
33. Here	Aquí	(ah-**kee**)
34. There	Allí	(ah-**yee**)

9. USEFUL MEDICAL WORDS

1. Wound	Herida	(ehr-**ee**-dah)
2. Bandage	vendaje	(vehn-**deh**-heh)
3. Sutures	Las suturas	(lahs soo-**toor**-ahs)
4. Stitches	Los puntos	(lohs **poon**-tohs)
5. Local anesthetic	Anestesia local	(ahn-ehs-tee-**see**-ah loh-**kahl**)
6. Thermometer	Termómetro	(tehr-**moh**-mehn-troh)
7. Temperature	Temperatura	(tehm-pehr-ah-**too**-rah)
8. Degrees	Grados	(**grah**-dohs)
9. Infection	Infección	(een-fehk-see-**ohn**)
10. A cold	Un resfriado	(oon rehs-free-**ah**-doh)
11. The flu	La gripe	(lah **gree**-peh)
12. Pneumonia	Neumonía	(neh-oo-mohn-**ee**-ah)
13. Treatment	Tratamiento	(trah-tah-mee-**ehn**-toh)
14. Antibiotics	Antibióticos	(ahn-tee-bee-**oh**-tee-kohs)
15. Appointment	Cita	(**see**-tah)
16. Pharmacy	Farmacia	(fahr-mah-**see**-ah)
17. Fracture	Fractura	(frahk-**too**-rah)
18. The bone is broken	El hueso está roto	(ehl oo-**eh**-soh ehs-**tah roh**-toh)
19. Burn	Quemadura	(keh-mah-**doo**-rah)
20. You can change clothes in this room	Puede cambiarse las ropas en este cuarto	(poo-**eh**-deh kahm-bee-**ahr**-seh las **roh**-pahs ehn ehs-teh koo-**ahr**-toh)

21.	Take off your shirt and pants	Quitese su camisa y pantalones	(kee-**teh**-seh soo kah-**mee**-sah ee pahn-tah-**lohn**-ehs)
22.	Put on this gown	Póngase esta bata	(**pohn**-gah-seh ehs-tah **bah**-tah)

10. MENTAL STATUS EXAM

1.	Do you know where you are?	¿Sabe usted dónde está?	(**sah**-beh oos-**tehd dohn**-deh ehs-**tah**)
2.	You are in a hospital	Usted está en un hospital	(oos-**tehd** ehs-**tah** ehn oon ohs-pee-**tahl**)
3.	What is today's date?	¿Cuál es la fecha de hoy?	(koo-**ahl** ehs lah **feh**-chah deh oy)
4.	Who is the president?	¿Quién es el presidente de los Estados Unidos?	(kee-**ehn** ehs ehl preh-see-**dehn**-teh deh lohs eh-**stah**-dohs oo-**nee**-dohs)
5.	Can you remember the names of 4 cities?	¿Puede recordar los nombres de cuatro ciudades?	(poo-**eh**-deh reh-kohr-**dahr** lohs **nohm**-bres de koo-**ah**-troh see-oo-**dah**-dehs)
6.	Chicago, Los Angeles, Dallas, Miami	Chicago, Los Angeles, Dallas, Miami	(chee-**kah**-goh, lohs ahn-**heh**-lehs, **dahl**-ahs mee-**ahm**-ee)
7.	What is 100 minus seven?	¿Cuánto es cien menos siete?	(koo-**ahn**-toh ehs see-**ehn meh**-nohs see-**eh**-teh)
8.	Do you feel nervous?	¿Siente nervios?	(see-**ehn**-teh nehr-**vee**-ohs)
9.	Do you feel it in your chest, abdomen, knees, and throat?	¿Lo siente en su pecho, abdomen, rodillas, y garganta?	(loh see-**ehn**-teh ehn soo **peh**-choh, ahb-**doh**-mehn, roh-**dee**-yahs, ee gahr-**gahn**-tah)

10. Do you feel sad?	¿Se siente triste?	(seh see-**ehn**-teh **trees**-teh)
11. Do you have difficulty eating?	¿Tiene dificultad comiendo?	(tee-**ehn**-eh dee-fee-kool-**tahd** koh-mee-**ehn**-doh)
12. And sleeping?	¿Y durmiendo?	(ee door-mee-**ehn**-doh)
13. Do you want to kill yourself?	¿Quiere suicidarse?	(kee-**ehr**-eh soo-ee-see-**dahr**-seh)

11. PRONUNCIATION

Spanish Letter	Like English	Example	Pronunciation
1. a	"ah" in fAther	cama (bed)	(**kah**-mah)
2. e	"eh" in bEd	tres (three)	(trehs)
3. i	"ee" in mEEt	si (yes)	(see)
4. o	"oh" in lOw	ocho (eight)	(**oh**-choh)
5. u	"oo" in flU	mucho (much/many)	(**moo**-choh)
6. y	"ee" in mEEt	y (and)	(ee)
7. h	h is silent	hijo (son)	(**ee**-hoh)
8. j	"h" in Hat	ojo (eye)	(**oh**-hoh)
9. qu	"k" in keep	que (what)	(keh)

12. QUESTION WORDS

It is important for you to learn the following question words. They will be extremely helpful to you because after you have learned them, you can ask questions. The medical questions in the booklet are structured to elicit "yes/no," numerical responses and other single-word or short-phrase answers so you will be able to understand answers from your patients.

1.	Who?	¿Quién?	(kee-**ehn**)
	Who is your doctor?	¿Quién es su doctor?	(kee-**ehn** ehs soo dohk-**tohr**)
2.	What?	¿Qué?	(**keh**)
	What medicines are you taking?	¿Qué medicinas toma?	(**keh** meh-dee-**see**-nahs **toh**-mah)
3.	When?	¿Cuándo?	(koo-**ahn**-doh)
	When did the pain start?	¿Cuándo comenzó el dolor?	(koo-**ahn**-doh koh-mee-ehn-**soh** ehl doh-**lohr**)
	When was your last menstrual period?	¿Cuándo fue su última regla?	(koo-**ahn**-doh foo-eh soo **ool**-tee-mah **reh**-glah)
4.	Where?	¿Dónde?	(**dohn**-deh)
	Where does it hurt?	¿Dónde le duele?	(**dohn**-deh leh doo-**eh**-leh)
5.	Why?	¿Porqué?	(pohr-**keh**)
	Why did you have a cesarean section?	¿Porqué tuvo cesárea?	(pohr-**keh too**-voh sehs-**sahr**-ee-ah)
6.	How?	¿Cómo?	(**koh**-moh)
	How are you?	¿Cómo está usted?	(**koh**-moh ehs-**tah** oos-**tehd**)
	How are you feeling?	¿Cómo se siente?	(**koh**-moh seh see-**ehn**-teh)
7.	How much/how many?	¿Cuántos?	(koo-**ahn**-tohs)
	How old are you?	¿Cuántos años tiene?	(koo-**ahn**-tohs **ah**-nyohs tee-**eh**-neh)
	How many times have you been pregnant?	¿Cuántas veces ha estado embarazada?	(koo-**ahn**-tohs **veh**-sehs ah ehs-**tah**-doh ehm-bahr-ah-**sah**-dah)
8.	Do you have?	¿Tiene?	(tee-**ehn**-eh)
	Do you have diabetes?	¿Tiene diabetes?	(tee-**ehn**-eh **dee**-ah-beh-tehs)
9.	Have you had?	¿Ha tenido?	(ah teh-**nee**-doh)
	Have you had an x-ray?	¿Ha tenido una radiografía?	(ah teh-**nee**-doh oon-ah rah-dee-oh-grah-**fee**-ah)
10.	Did you have?	¿Tuvo?	(**too**-voh)
	Did you have a heart attack?	¿Tuvo un ataque al corazón?	(**too**-voh oon ah-**tah**-keh ahl kohr-ah-**sohn**)

13. VERB CONJUGATION

The three most important tenses for Medical Spanish are the present (present indicative), future, and command form. The conjugation of a verb is the same for the he, she, you (el, ella, usted) pronouns. Therefore you should learn these three tenses for the "he-she-you" pronoun. This is all you need in terms of verb conjugation for the vast majority of situations. The past tense is occasionally helpful.

REGULAR VERBS

Verb	Past (preterit)	Present (indicative)	Future	Command
Tomar *(to take, to eat, or to drink)*				
I		Tomo	Tomaré	
he/she/you (sing)	Tomó	Toma	Tomará	Tome
we		Tomamos	Tomaremos	
they (m,f), you (pl)	Tomaron	Toman	Tomarán	Tomen

Verb	Past (preterit)	Present (indicative)	Future	Command
Deber *(to owe, must, should)*				
I		debo	deberé	
he/she/you (sing)	debió	debe	deberá	deba
we		debemos	deberemos	
they (m,f), you (pl)	debieron	deben	deberán	deban

Verb	Past (preterit)	Present (indicative)	Future	Command
Escribir *(to write)*				
I		Escribo	Escribiré	
he/she/you (sing)	Escribió	Escribe	Escribirá	Escriba
we		Escribimos	Escribiremos	
they (m,f), you (pl)	Escribieron	Escriben	Escribirán	Escriban

14. PATIENT REPLIES

1. Yes	Si	(see)
2. No	No	(noh)
3. Better	Mejor	(meh-**hohr**)
4. Worse	Peor	(peh-**ohr**)
5. Same	Lo mismo	(loh **mees**-moh)
6. Ask my wife	Pregunta a mi esposa	(preh-**goon**-tah ah mee eh-**spoh**-sah)
7. I don't know	No sé	(noh **seh**)
8. I do not understand	No entiendo	(noh ehn-tee-**ehn**-doh)
9. When can I eat?	¿Cuándo puedo comer?	(koo-**ahn**-doh poo-**eh**-doh koh-**mehr**)
10. When can I go home?	¿Cuándo puede salir?	(koo-**ahn**-doh poo-**eh**-deh sah-**lehr**)
11. Can you give me medicine for the pain?	¿Puede darme más medicina para aliviar el dolor?	(poo-**eh**-deh **dahr**-meh **mahs** meh-dee-**see**-nah pah-rah ah-lee-vee-**ahr** ehl doh-**lohr**)

15. CASSETTE CONTENTS

Page numbers in parentheses below are the beginning text pages for cassette contents.

SIDE 1 (30 MINUTES)

SIDE 2 (29.42 MINUTES)